POSTURAL AND RELAXATION TRAINING

IN PHYSIOTHERAPY AND PHYSICAL EDUCATION

JOHN H. C. COLSON

F.C.S.P., F.S.R.G., M.A.O.T.

*Former Director of Rehabilitation, Pinderfields General Hospital, and sometime
Principal, School of Remedial Gymnastics and Recreational Therapy*

Foreword by

J. M. P. CLARK

M.B.E., M.B., Ch.B., F.R.C.S.

SECOND EDITION

WILLIAM HEINEMANN · MEDICAL BOOKS · LTD
LONDON

First published 1956
Second edition 1968

© John H. C. Colson, 1968

SBN 433 06300 9

Printed in Great Britain by
The Whitefriars Press Ltd., London and Tonbridge

FOREWORD

Mr. Colson has a very long experience as a teacher, and his outstanding quality in this capacity is clarity of exposition. He has already given sufficient evidence of his academic attainments in the previous books he has published, and this has been recognized officially by the reception with which his books have been accorded. In this small volume the author has set out once more to clear the air and give light on a subject which has long been hampered by shibboleths. He will have contributed in no small measure in this way to the slow death of obsolete ideas on posture and postural training when his book has been read by the large number of people to whom it will inevitably make a strong appeal.

In this book is succinctly set out the conception of posture as held by the modern orthopaedic surgeon, and the account is mercifully not encumbered by a speculative and nebulous theoretical background to detract from its straightforward approach. The vocabulary of exercise therapy is sufficiently lucid for even a medical man to comprehend, and it will be a godsend to the physiotherapist, remedial gymnast and physical educationist. When it is recalled that Mr. Colson has been responsible for the training of by far the greater part of the remedial gymnasts in this country, that he has had a profound effect on many physiotherapists and occupational therapists direct (and indirectly on a great many more through his writings), and that his work is well recognized in the field of physical education, it is obvious that he speaks with authority and that he will be listened to with profit.

The author has written nothing in this book of which he has not had personal experience. It follows therefore that the book is primarily a practical manual which is the fruit of clinical and teaching experience. In eschewing the fog of didactic debate, and the metaphysical miasma commonly associated with books and teaching on the fringe of medical subjects (and consequently the source of much bewilderment to the student), Mr. Colson will be rewarded by the appreciation of an increasing number of disciples whose path will be the narrow, straight one of modesty and understanding in the face of the vast uncertainty of scientific medicine. It only remains for me to wish this little guide and its author all the success they so richly deserve.

JOHN M. P. CLARK.

PREFACE TO THE SECOND EDITION

In preparing the new edition of this book I have revised and expanded the text, particularly in the sections dealing with posture, and included a chapter on the prevention of back strain. I have also added a chapter on balance exercises and techniques as applied to postural training.

As before, the book is intended as a guide to the methods used to-day in the treatment of postural defects and the various conditions for which relaxation therapy is prescribed. The theoretical background of postural and relaxation training has been covered, but the main emphasis of the book is on the practical aspects of the work.

The account of the various types of postural defects is based on the teaching of the late Mr. Philip Wiles, Orthopaedic Surgeon Emeritus, The Middlesex Hospital. The original account was written under his guidance, and it is a very great pleasure—if a sad duty—to record my grateful appreciation for all his help. His work was to me, as to so many others, an inspiration.

I must acknowledge my indebtedness to the late Mrs. Helen Heardman, M.C.S.P., who first interested me in the postural training methods which I have described here, and was so generous in imparting her knowledge and skill.

I must thank Mr. J. M. P. Clark, Orthopaedic Surgeon at the General Infirmary at Leeds, for writing the Foreword and for his constant encouragement and advice. I must also thank Dr. Maurice Parsonage, Consultant Physician to the Neurological Department in the General Infirmary at Leeds, for his chapter on psychosomatic tension states. This section of the book will be of great value to those who are asked to give relaxation training for these conditions.

My thanks are due also to Mr. W. J. Armour, M.C.S.P., M.S.R.G., Principal of the School of Remedial Gymnastics and Recreational Therapy, Pinderfields General Hospital, for his helpful criticism and advice. I must also thank Mr. G. Sommerville, M.S.R.G., Senior Remedial Gymnast in the School Health Service, Derby Education Committee, for the help he has given me in assessing and testing out some of the postural training techniques.

Thanks are also due to the following: the publishers who have so generously allowed me to quote from various textbooks, particularly J. and A. Churchill Ltd., who allowed me to reproduce the illustrations of the postural defects from Wiles's and Sweetnam's *Essentials of Orthopaedics*; the artist, Mr. S. Francis, whose drawings help to explain the text so well. I must also thank Mr. Owen R. Evans, Managing Director, William Heinemann Medical Books Ltd., for his encouragement and continued interest in the book.

JOHN H. C. COLSON.

March, 1968.

CONTENTS

PART ONE: POSTURAL TRAINING

Chapter 1

THE MECHANICS OF POSTURE

The posture of normal individuals varies considerably and is influenced by such factors as body build, personality, habits and occupation.

To maintain the upright posture the muscles on each side of the joints concerned work in a state of balanced isometric contraction. Although practically every muscle and joint in the body is involved, fatigue is reduced to a minimum, because the number of fibres employed simultaneously in each muscle is relatively small, and there is a constant change of contracting fibres. The whole process is controlled by the central nervous system, which receives afferent impulses from the muscles, eyes, ears and skin and—after integrating them with the habits of stance and movement of the particular individual concerned—translates the information received into efferent motor impulses.

The part played by the ligaments in maintaining posture is controversial. Some argue that the strength, structure and general arrangement of the ligaments makes it obvious that it is an important part. The majority of authorities, however, disagree with this view. Clark says: "Ligaments are largely responsible for the stability of joints and they act as checks to the range of movement in a joint in any particular direction, but they were never intended to withstand continued stress. Ligaments are only slightly extensible, they are tough, they are easily ruptured, and they have a nerve supply. Undue stress on ligaments is prevented by muscle control, but should this action break down or become inadequate, the stress on the ligaments results in strain, which is denoted as pain. Chronic strain eventually causes ligaments to stretch with consequent distortion of bone and joint, and with functional collapse of the affected part, as is so well exemplified in the feet of obese people." [1]

For these reasons ligaments can play no direct part in maintaining posture. "Their function is complementary to that of the muscles; the muscles cause movements and maintain posture within the ordinary range, whereas the ligaments limit the extremes of movement and take the strain when the muscles are fatigued or overloaded." [2]

Body image. The posture of an individual is best considered in relation to the concept of "body image" put forward by Henry Head to convey the idea each person has of his own body. "It is a very personal affair which is constructed from information derived from intrinsic sources and related to the environment, both objective and subjective. The principal intrinsic sources are visual impulses, tactile impulses and proprioceptive impulses. Visual information about ourselves is peculiar in that we see ourselves, for the most part, either in reflection, or else upside down; we relate it to the right-way-up appearance of other people. Tactile impulses tell us what we feel like, and this is different from the feel of others because it is felt simultaneously by both the touching and the touched parts of the body. Proprioception is perhaps the most important of these percepts. It is entirely personal without possibility of relation to the experience of others, and it is unconscious. It gives information about the movements of joints and the relative length of the controlling muscles, hence of position in space.

"The body image develops slowly from earliest childhood and changes continuously during growth. Not only is the personality developing, but also the values of the information derived from proprioceptive impulses are constantly changing. Growth of the limbs and trunk is induced entirely through the agency of the bones. Bones have an intrinsic power of growth in length, whereas the soft tissues—periosteum, muscle, tendon, fascia and skin— grow in length only in response to the 'stretching' effect of the growing bone. The proprioceptive information derived from these tissues must, therefore, require continual adjustment to yield accurate information as to posture." [3]

During growth the mental record of the body pattern (or "schema" as Head termed it) is constantly being modified. In other words, the postural reflexes are subject to continual adjustment. When growth ceases the posture becomes relatively stable. Even then, however, it may be changed by some modification in personality or physique.

To sum up: the essential requirements for a good posture in a

normal healthy body are adequate muscles and correctly condi-
tioned reflexes.

Posture of the Hip Joint

In the erect position the posture of the hip joint is the key to
the posture of the whole body. This is because the hip posture
determines (*a*) the angle of the antero-posterior inclination of
the pelvis (the pelvic tilt), and (b) the degree of rotation of the
legs, and therefore the posture of the feet.[4]

The pelvis is balanced on the femoral heads, and forms the
foundation upon which the spinal column is erected. Any change
in the antero-posterior inclination of the pelvis causes a corresponding change in the position of the 5th lumbar vertebra which,
in turn, alters the posture of the spine as a whole,* as shown in
Figs. 2–5, pp. 9–11.

Control of the antero-posterior pelvic inclination is exercised
ordinarily by the hip muscles, and it is only in unusual circumstances that it becomes a function of the muscles of the trunk.
The inclination is increased by contraction of the hip flexors, and
decreased by contraction of the hip extensors, i.e. the glutei,
hamstrings and posterior adductors.

Wiles stresses that the three glutei function in one unit as part
of the extensor group of muscles that maintain the upright
position. "Their combined, unapposed action, produces extension,
abduction, and lateral rotation of the hip joints, the thighs or
pelvis being moved according to which is free. Postural increase
in the length of the glutei allows the pelvis to tilt forwards and
the femora to rotate medially." [5]

Rotation of the hip joints, with the knees extended and the
feet in firm contact with the floor, affects the position of the feet,
as previously indicated. Lateral rotation causes inversion of the
foot and a raising of the medial longitudinal arch, while medial
rotation (brought about in certain postural defects by a general
slump of the anti-gravity muscles) produces eversion of the foot
and a lowering of the medial longitudinal arch (Fig. 7, p. 14). This
is because the lower leg rotates with the thigh, and the talus is
held securely in the mortice of the ankle joint; hip rotation,
therefore, has a direct passive effect on the sub-talar and mid-
tarsal joints.

* A lateral tilt of the pelvis at one hip also produces a corresponding change
in the position of the spine (*see* Fig. 55, p. 60).

When the medial longitudinal arch is raised by lateral rotation of the hip joint, the tendency for the head of the first metatarsal bone to lift from the floor is counteracted by the action of the peroneus longus muscle; the tibialis posterior muscle also works to maintain the medial longitudinal arch in its corrected position.

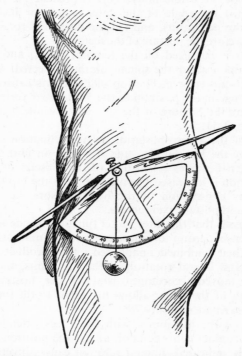

FIG. 1a. Measuring the pelvic inclination with the Wiles's pelvic inclinometer. Cf. Fig. 1b, opposite.

Measuring the pelvic inclination. For comparative purposes it is useful to be able to measure the angle of the antero-posterior tilt of the pelvis. Wiles [6] has described a simple and practical way of doing this with the pelvic inclinometer illustrated in Fig. 1. His method uses arbitrary points selected because they are easily palpable; it is quick and sufficiently accurate.

One blade of the inclinometer is placed on the upper border of the symphysis pubis, and the other is placed on a mark made in the mid-line at the level of the posterior superior iliac spines. The plumb bob is adjusted so that it is parallel with the calibrated scale plate and a reading is taken (Fig. 1a). The pelvic inclination measured by this method averages 31° in males and 28° in females. Variations up to 4° on each side of the average are within the "normal" range.

It should be noted that the pelvis is more horizontal in infants, and the inclination increases steadily with growth. "At four years

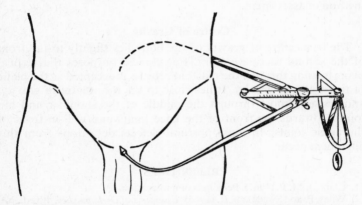

FIG. 1b. Measuring the angle of pelvic tilt. One blade of the pelvic inclinometer is placed on the upper border of the symphysis pubis, and the other is placed on a mark made in the mid-line at the level of the posterior superior iliac spines. The plumb bob is adjusted so that it is parallel with the calibrated scale plate and a reading is taken.

of age it is about 22° in both sexes, and at seven years 25°. The adult angle of inclination is reached about the tenth or eleventh year when the variation due to sex first appears." [7]

When a pelvic inclinometer is not available two other methods of measuring the pelvic inclination may be used. They are both based on the assumption that the pelvic tilt is "normal" in the standing position when (a) the symphysis pubis and the anterior superior iliac spines lie in the same vertical plane, and (b) an imaginary line drawn through the symphysis pubis and the lumbosacral angle forms an angle of between 50° and 60° with a horizontal line.

Assessment of Antero-posterior Curves of the Spine

The curves of the spine, when viewed from the side, may be extremely difficult to assess, particularly if they are masked by subcutaneous fat or an increased development of the erector spinae muscles. If the sacrum is placed more horizontally than usual the gluteal masses are more prominent, and the lumbar curve appears to be increased. When the scapulae are placed rather forward the dorsal curve appears to be more pronounced. Wiles considers that radiography provides the only accurate method of assessment.

Centre of Gravity

The true centre of gravity of the body lies slightly to the front of the second sacral vertebra. For clinical purposes the vertical plane passing through the mastoid process is accepted as the plane of the centre of gravity. It lies close to the true centre of gravity, and passes almost through the middle of the shoulder and hip joints, towards the front of the knee joints and well in front of the ankle joints. In most postural defects deviations from this alignment occur.

REFERENCES

1. Clark, J. M. P. (1967). Personal communication.
2. Wiles, P. and Sweetnam, R. (1965), *Essentials of Orthopaedics*, 4th ed., p.1. London: J. and A. Churchill Ltd.
3. Wiles, P. and Sweetnam, R. (1965), *ibid*, pp. 2 and 3.
4. Wiles, P. and Sweetnam, R. (1965), *ibid*, p. 6.
5. Wiles, P. and Sweetnam, R. (1965), *ibid*, p. 8.
6. Wiles, P. and Sweetnam, R. (1965), *ibid*, p. 6.
7. Wiles, P. and Sweetnam, R. (1965), *ibid*, p. 6.

Chapter 2

POSTURAL DEFECTS

Aetiology

Postural defects may be considered as variations from the accepted normal posture; they can be corrected by active muscular effort on the part of the patient. Generally the entire posture of the body is affected, and it is unusual to find only one part of the body involved. For example, valgus feet are frequently associated with defects of the antero-posterior curves of the spine.

"Postural defects occur when the postural reflexes do not conform with the accepted standards. The defects arise most often during periods of rapid growth and at times of emotional uncertainty. It is seldom easy to be sure of the precise cause in a particular child, but occasionally it is clear, for example when there is an upset in general well-being as occurs in the undernourished, or in toxaemia due to chronic infection. Nor are the psychological factors usually obvious because the emotional disturbance is seldom gross and more often there is only some minor maladjustment.

"Children have much to learn and tend to concentrate on one aspect of life at a time. Whilst a young child is busily enquiring about the many phenomena surrounding him, and being well satisfied with the mobility given by his recently acquired powers of locomotion, he is unlikely to care much about the way his body functions. But at a later period, perhaps when games have interested him, he will all unconsciously attend to the defects of the body that may have developed meanwhile. Girls in their early teens frequently stand badly and are ungainly in their movements; it is noticeable that the age at which they correct themselves often corresponds with the first display of real interest in the other sex.

"Gross psychological disturbances occasionally appear to be responsible for the development of postural defects, and it does seem possible to make a direct correlation between the emotional and the physical condition. An extreme example is seen in the 'depressed' child who has become profoundly discouraged in his attempts to cope with a difficult environment; mentally he is tired, bodily he has given way to gravity and has a sagging jaw and drooping eyelids, rounded shoulders, a tilted pelvis and flat feet. The mental and physical conditions go together, and any attempt to change the physical condition until such time as the psychological adjustment has been improved leads to disappointment.

"The 'anxious' child, on the other hand, is actively struggling with his difficulties. The picture is of a hypersensitive, alarmed child, perhaps subject to nightmares, and sometimes with a stammer. Physically he tends to have valgus feet, knock-knees, and round shoulders—a position of fear—but in contrast with the 'depressive', his muscles are tense rather than slack. Again, the 'obsessional' child may have queer habits of gait and posture, often asymmetrical, which are impossible to explain except in association with the psychological condition. Most patients do not, however, show so extreme a picture, and the correlation between the physical and psychological findings is seldom obvious." [1]

In the past it was customary to lay the blame for some postural defects on the immediate surroundings of the child, such as bad school furniture, and the type of clothing. Wiles says: "It is difficult to believe that such factors are of great importance; a child who is going to sit badly will do so at any desk, and it would be far more rational to blame a boring lesson that fails to hold his attention." [2]

TYPES OF POSTURAL DEFECTS OF THE SPINE

Postural defects of the spine may be divided into two main groups: (1) Defects of the antero-posterior curves of the spine (Figs. 2–5, pp. 9–11), and (2) Postural lateral curvature, or postural scoliosis (Fig. 6, p. 11).

Defects of the Antero-posterior curves

This group includes: (a) Lumbar lordosis, (b) Sway back, (c) Flat back, and (d) Round back. In analyzing the mechanics of these defects it must be remembered that in order to maintain the upright posture the centre of gravity of the whole body must be kept above the area occupied by the feet.

The following notes on the individual defects have been based on descriptions given in *Essentials of Orthopaedics*.[3] In these descriptions, to make the mechanics clear, it is assumed that the pelvic inclination alters first, and then movements of the rest of the body are made afterwards to adjust the centre of gravity. In fact, the defects are brought about by a gradual "slumping" process, and not by separate movements.

Lumbar lordosis (Fig. 2). The pelvis tilts forward and the spine follows its movement. To bring the centre of gravity above the feet the patient extends the lumbar spine and so increases its concavity (Fig. 2). Frequently there is an associated dorsal

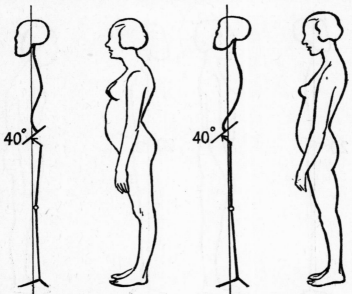

FIG. 2. Lumbar lordosis.

After P. Wiles's and R. Sweetnam's 'Essentials of Orthopaedics', 4th Edition, J. & A. Churchill Ltd.

FIG. 3. Sway back.

After P. Wiles's and R. Sweetnam's 'Essentials of Orthopaedics', 4th Edition, J. & A. Churchill Ltd.

kyphosis, with rounding of the shoulders, medially-rotated hip joints and valgus feet. This is due to a general slump of the anti-gravity muscles.

Sway back. (Fig. 3). The pelvis is tilted forward, but the lumbar spine lacks mobility and cannot compensate by the production of a complete lumbar lordosis, as previously des-cribed, because of an associated thoracolumbar kyphosis (*see* over). The lumbar spine is therefore bent backward sharply at the lumbosacral angle, and the centre of gravity is kept above the feet by the legs being allowed to incline slightly forward from the ankle joints, so that the pelvis is carried forward (Fig. 3). There is also a general slump of the anti-gravity muscles with the associated round shoulders, medially rotated hips and valgus feet.

Thoracolumbar kyphosis. "This is a very common localized form of adolescent kyphosis in which the bodies of the lower thoracic and upper lumbar vertebrae become slightly wedge-

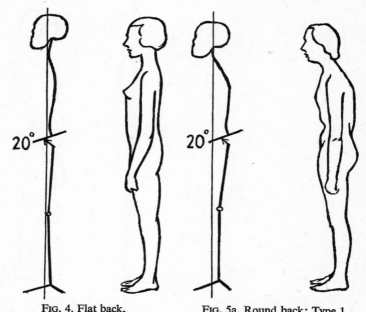

FIG. 4. Flat back.

After P. Wiles's and R. Sweetnam's 'Essentials of Orthopaedics', 4th Edition, J. & A. Churchill Ltd.

FIG. 5a. Round back: Type 1.

After P. Wiles's and R. Sweetnam's 'Essentials of Orthopaedics', 4th Edition, J. & A. Churchill Ltd.

shaped. The condition commonly accompanies certain postural defects, and possibly is caused by them. The abnormal posture increases the stress on the anterior portions of the vertebral bodies and intervertebral discs, and this may interfere with their development. The thoracolumbar region, where the alteration in curve from concave to convex makes it mechanically weaker than the rest of the spine, is the site where such changes occur most frequently." [4]

Flat back (Fig. 4, p. 10). The pelvic inclination decreases and the "normal" concavity of the lumbar spine is flattened out (Fig. 4). This type of defect, if allowed to go uncorrected, leads to the development of a stiff spine in later life, with intractable backache. Personal observation suggests that flat back is often associated with congenital shortening of the hamstrings.

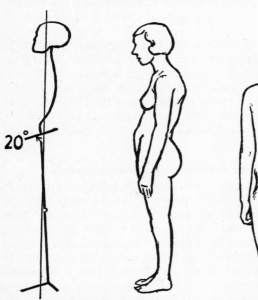

FIG. 5b. Round back: Type 2.

After P. Wiles's and R. Sweetnam's 'Essentials of Orthopaedics', 4th Edition, J. & A. Churchill Ltd.

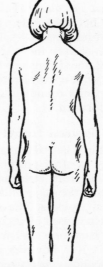

FIG. 6. Postural lateral curvature or postural scoliosis.

After P. Wiles's and R. Sweetnam's 'Essentials of Orthopaedics', 4th Edition, J. & A. Churchill Ltd.

Children with a reduced lumbar curve are often thought by their parents, and others, to have a "lovely stance" and a "wonderful straight back". The parents are frequently "put out" when the fault is explained, and often take a lot of convincing before they will co-operate.

Round back (Figs. 5a and 5b). This is not such a clearly defined group. The pelvic inclination is decreased and is associated with thoracolumbar kyphosis (p. 10). Figs. 5a and 5b indicate the ways in which the body compensates for the defect. In the first (Fig. 5a), "which gives the name to the group, the trunk is bent forwards in the lower lumbar region reducing the lumbar curve. The legs are inclined slightly backwards at the ankles and the great trochanters are behind the mastoid line." [5] In the second way (Fig. 5b) "the mechanism is very similar to that in sway back. The legs are inclined forwards and the trunk backwards causing a low lumbar angulation, and the great trochanters are in front of the mastoid line." [5]

Round shoulders. The defect seldom exists alone as a clinical entity, but constitutes part of a general postural defect (*see* Lumbar lordosis, p. 9). It occurs when the transverse back muscles, which link the scapulae with the spine, allow them to slip forward and downward by the action of gravity. The position of the scapulae is exaggerated by the slight kyphosis which generally accompanies round shoulders, and by the head and neck being poked forward.

Postural Lateral Curvature or Postural Scoliosis

"Postural lateral curvature is a disorder in function of a similar etiology to other postural deformities. It is an entirely different condition from structural scoliosis; it is not associated with changes in the shape of the vertebrae, and it can be fully corrected by voluntary effort. The older surgeons, who believed that scoliosis was often caused by occupational habits, concluded that postural lateral curvature was frequently transformed into a structural scoliosis. It is, however, doubtful if this ever occurs . . . The very word scoliosis has a serious significance in the minds of both laymen and doctors; since postural lateral curvature has a different etiology and a different prognosis, it is better not to classify it with scoliosis, but to include it with postural defects where it properly belongs.

"Postural curvature is seen chiefly in adolescents, and in girls more often than boys. There is a smooth curve without sharp angulation, and it is convex to the left more frequently than to the right. Fig. 6. It usually includes all the lumbar and thoracic vertebrae, the apex being in the mid- or upper thoracic region (total scoliosis). Rotation of the vertebrae, if any, is slight, and it is not fixed; there is no deformity of the ribs, such as occurs invariably in structural scoliosis.

"The curve is abolished by flexing the spine, by standing on one leg, or by any similar movement that involves synergic contraction of the erector spinae. Frequently, but not always, it disappears when sitting, and when standing it can usually be corrected by voluntary muscular effort.

"The prognosis in children is excellent because the probability is that the curvature will correct spontaneously. The defect is often an indication that all is not well with the child's general health or emotional adjustment, but when these are satisfactory correction is easily achieved.

"Postural lateral curvature seldom persists from adolescence to adult life. An adult with such a curve is likely to have acquired it freshly; it may then be the result of bodily or mental fatigue and will require treating accordingly." [6]

DEFECTS OF THE LOWER LIMBS
Postural Pes Valgus (Postural "Flat Foot")

Of this condition Wiles states: "A valgus, pronated, or 'flat-footed', posture of the feet developing during childhood or early adolescence is usually postural in origin. The postural nature of the defect can usually be demonstrated by instructing the patient to rotate the legs laterally while the feet are kept parallel on the ground until the patellae face directly forwards; this will restore the shape of the feet to normal. Fig. 7b.

"Postural defects of the feet seldom occur in isolation. They are nearly always associated with postural defects of the antero-posterior curves of the spine, particularly those in which the pelvic inclination is increased, i.e. lumbar lordosis and sway back. This is because the gluteal muscles are lateral rotators as well as extensors of the hips and consequently, when there is a general slump of the anti-gravity muscles allowing the pelvis to rotate forwards, the legs rotate medially at the same time. The feet do not move with the legs or they would point inwards, but instead their posture is changed by a rotatory movement in such a way that the longitudinal arches disappear." [7] Fig. 7a. See also Posture of Hip Joint, p. 3.

Genu valgum or Knock-knees

Genu valgum is extremely common in infancy—so common, in fact, that it can hardly be regarded as abnormal. It nearly always corrects itself spontaneously.

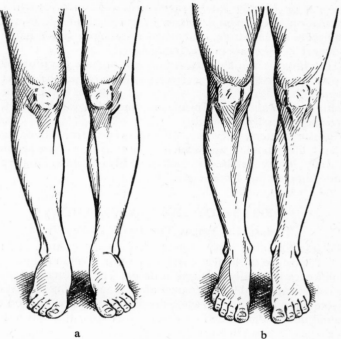

a   b

FIG. 7. (*a*) Postural pes valgus (postural "flat foot"). A general slump of the anti-gravity muscles permits the pelvis to rotate forwards, increasing its inclination, and the legs to rotate medially, thus twisting the feet into the valgus position. Note that the patellae face medially.

(*b*) Correction of the foot defect by lateral rotation of the hips joints. The patellae now face forwards.

"Knock-knees in young children, at any rate in Great Britain where florid rickets is now uncommon, is usually of the 'idiopathic' type. It is caused by growth at the lateral side of the epiphyseal disc at the lower end of the femur proceeding rather more slowly than that at the medial side. The line of the knee joint therefore slopes slightly laterally instead of being horizontal. In a large majority, growth at the lateral side eventually catches up with the medial, and the defect rights itself spontaneously. The reason for this irregularity in growth is quite unknown." [8]

Valgus feet are often associated with the more severe degrees of knock-knees, particularly in heavy children. Frequently there is an associated poor general posture, with medial rotation of the legs. The valgus position of the feet occurs partly because of this, and partly because of pressure on the medial borders.

The foot condition generally recovers spontaneously as the legs become straight. If the medial rotation of the legs persists postural training is required, as indicated on p. 35.

Wiles considers that as "idiopathic" genu valgum nearly always recovers spontaneously, all treatment is of doubtful value. He says that the only conservative measure available is to wedge the medial sides of the heels and soles of the shoes with the object of relieving the strain on the medial sides of the knees. Exercises have no effect on the deformity.[9]

Genu varum or Bow legs

Bow legs may be grouped into two main groups: Real and Apparent.[10] The first group includes deformities caused by rickets and tibia vara, and those occurring in infancy. The second group includes deformities caused by medial rotation of the hips and obliquity of the ankle joints.

Bow legs due to rickets and tibia vara are not considered here, as their treatment is outside the scope of this book.

Bow legs in infancy. The majority of babies are, for a time, bow-legged. The site of the bowing is difficult to assess, but is probably at the knees, and may be caused by bulky nappies increasing the pressure on the medial sides of the epiphyses of the femora and tibiae. The legs straighten spontaneously over a period of time, provided there is no general disease or structural defect present, and treatment is not required.

Apparent bow legs. Apparent bow legs in older children and young adults is usually caused by faulty posture. The bow-legged appearance is brought about by medial rotation of the legs, associated with some degree of hyper-extension of the knees (genu recurvatum). When the hips are rotated laterally, as described on p. 35, the bow-legged appearance is eliminated. Postural treatment, as described on p. 36, is possible only during childhood and adolescence.

Apparent bow legs can also be produced by obliquity of the ankle joints. This is a temporary defect of growth in which the lower articular surfaces of the tibiae sometimes fail to develop evenly, and slope a little medially instead of being parallel with the ground.

Spontaneous correction generally takes place during growth, but a small degree of deformity remains; this may cause slightly valgus feet. There is little point in using physical treatment for the foot condition, and surgery is required only on rare occasions.

REFERENCES

1. Wiles, P. and Sweetnam, R. (1965), *Essentials of Orthopaedics*, 4th ed., p. 5. London: J. and A. Churchill Ltd.
2. Wiles, P. and Sweetnam, R. (1965), *ibid*, p. 4.
3. Wiles, P. and Sweetnam, R. (1965), *ibid*, p. 10.
4. Wiles, P. and Sweetnam, R. (1965), *ibid*, p. 9.
5. Wiles, P. and Sweetnam, R. (1965), *ibid*, p. 12.
6. Wiles, P. and Sweetnam, R. (1965), *ibid*, pp. 14 and 15.
7. Wiles, P. and Sweetnam, R. (1965), *ibid*, p. 18.
8. Wiles, P. and Sweetnam, R. (1965), *ibid*, p. 27.
9. Wiles, P. and Sweetnam, R. (1965), *ibid*, p. 27.
10. Wiles, P. and Sweetnam, R. (1965), *ibid*, p. 27.

CHAPTER 3

CORRECT STANDING AND SITTING

Before dealing with the practical aspects of postural training it is helpful to consider the basic features of a good standing and sitting position.

Standing (Fig. 8)

Feet. The feet point straight forward and are placed slightly apart, so as to provide a sound base. A distance of two to three finger-breadths between the heads of the first metatarsal bones gives the right amount of separation.

The weight of the body is taken evenly by the heel and the heads of the first and fifth metatarsal bones of each foot—the three points of bearing or contact of the foot [1]—the balls of the toes being pressed down against the floor or the shoe surface without the toes being flexed. The use of the intrinsic muscles in this action is of great value in stabilizing the feet.

Knee joints. The knees are extended, but not hyperextended.

Hip joints. The hip joints are held in the correct degree of extension and lateral rotation. This ensures that (*a*) the pelvic inclination is within the average range as described on p. 5, (*b*) the "normal" lumbar curve is unimpaired, and (*c*) the position of the legs is good, i.e. the patellae face directly forward (Fig. 7, p. 14).

Sub-costal angle. The sub-costal angle is held open as widely as possible without strain (Fig. 8*b*). Opening the sub-costal angle has the effect of decreasing the thoracic convexity (probably through the fixator action of the erector spinae muscles) without bringing about an extension of the lumbar spine.

Cervical spine. The neck is held as straight as possible without eradicating the "normal" cervical curve. The chin should be level, and there must be nothing forced or tense about the head and neck positions.

Scapulae and arms. The shoulders are held so that the scapulae are flat and the outer ends of the clavicles lie slightly further back than the inner ends. The shoulder joints are rotated laterally, with the olecranon processes facing backward; the radio-ulnar joints are held in a neutral position with the knuckles of the fingers facing outward.

The laterally-rotated position of the shoulder joints is normally associated with a good position of the scapulae. It is most im-

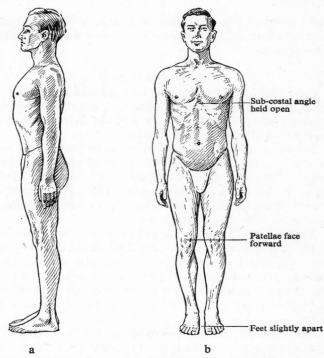

Sub-costal angle held open

Patellae face forward

Feet slightly apart

a   b

FIG. 8. Correct standing position. Once acquired there should be no suggestion of strain or tension about the posture.

portant to recognize that, although the knuckles may be facing outward, the shoulder joints may be rotated medially in an incorrect manner, with the radio-ulnar joints rotated laterally. "This permits winged shoulder blades, and is a thoroughly bad habit." [2]

Hands. The fingers are relaxed.

Avoidance of Strain

Once acquired there should be no suggestion of strain or tension about the correct standing posture. When the position is first taught and practised, however, some degree of strain is generally unavoidable. Most subjects, having taken up the correct position, find it helpful if they concentrate on reaching their full height without stretching or forcing themselves upward. "Come to your full height, but don't strain", is a useful coaching instruction.

Sitting (Figs. 9 and 10)

Hip and knee joints. Ideally the chair used should be an upright one with a firm flat seat. The seat should be of such a height that when the subject sits on it with the feet resting on the floor, the hip and knee joints are flexed to about 90°.

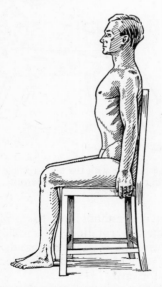

FIG. 9. Correct sitting position. The chair seat is of the right height for the subject, as it allows him to sit with his thighs well supported and his feet on the floor. If a chair with a lower seat is used the subject should sit as shown above, but with the knees slightly extended and the feet resting on the floor. Cf. Fig. 10, overleaf.

Thighs. The ischial tuberosities, and as much of the thighs as possible, are supported by the chair seat.

Pelvis. The posterior surface of the pelvis rests against the back of the chair, so that it is well supported.

Spine and Arms. The spine, head, arms and hands are held as described in the previous section on the standing posture.

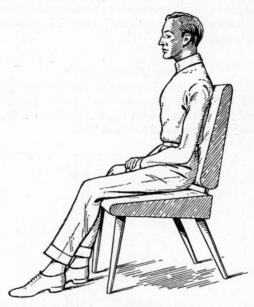

FIG. 10. A good sitting posture with the arms resting in a relaxed position, but the scapulae held correctly.

Once the subject understands how to correct the position of the scapulae by laterally rotating the shoulder joints, and can manage this with ease, he may let the hands rest on the thighs in a more "relaxed" attitude (Fig. 10), provided he does not allow the scapulae to slip forward.

Anchorage of the Pelvis

In the correct sitting position the pelvis is anchored securely. The rectus femoris and hamstring muscles exert a balanced pull on its upper and lower aspects from their insertion points on the legs. The legs are stabilized, as the feet rest flat on the floor.

When the back of the pelvis is without support, and the feet are drawn under the chair—a common enough posture—the pelvis is insecure. This may cause back strain and general fatigue of the trunk muscles.

REFERENCES

1. Dickson, F. D. and Diveley, R. L., *Functional Disorders of the Foot*, 3rd ed., p. 22. Philadelphia: J. B. Lippincott and Co.
2. McConnell, J. K. and Griffin, F. W. W. (1947), *Health and Muscular Habits*, 1st ed., pp. 44–53. London: J. and A. Churchill Ltd.

Chapter 4

POSTURAL TRAINING

SECTION 1: BASIC PRINCIPLES

To achieve good posture in patients suffering from postural defects it is necessary to establish new postural habits. In other words, the bad postural habits must be broken and *habitual* good habits of posture instituted.

The patient acquires the new sense of posture by constant practice of the correct position. He is trained to maintain the position while performing various exercises and while carrying out the ordinary movements of everyday life. It must be stressed that in themselves the exercises and movements are relatively unimportant; it is the way in which the body is held during their performance that matters. This fact is frequently misunderstood.

If limitation of mobility prevents full correction of the defects by voluntary effort (and usually this applies only to a small proportion of patients), the postural training must be supplemented by mobility exercises. Mobility is of particular importance where there is a thoracolumbar kyphosis (p. 10), or limitation of hip extension.

Mobility may be limited by contracted ligaments and joint capsules, and by "shortened" muscles; it can also be limited by structural changes in the shape of the vertebrae, as in thoracolumbar kyphosis. Mobility exercises of the right type are of considerable assistance in correcting the changes in the soft tissues; they are of no value whatever in cases where bony changes have occurred.

Exercises to strengthen the muscles which are used to counteract the postural defects are always useful. Strengthening the muscles helps to improve their efficiency.

Education in relaxation is also of value, as poor posture is sometimes associated with unnecessary muscular tension. Generally this tension occurs in the muscles of the shoulder girdle and the extensor muscles of the neck.

Systems of training. Many systems of postural correction

have been based on these principles. Some incorporate a background of physical education; others employ music and various forms of dancing, including classical ballet dancing and ball-room dancing. Wiles [1] states that the training for classical ballet dancing requires movements that are readily adapted for correcting postural defects. It gives poise and grace, and is excellent for musical children provided work on the "pointes" is excluded and extreme lateral rotation of the feet is excluded.

Co-operation of the patient. Success in postural training, whatever the system followed, depends on obtaining the full co-operation of the patient. This is often difficult when dealing with young children and some adolescents who have a "Couldn't care less" attitude towards the whole matter. Some parents also show little or no interest, or have insufficient intelligence to be of help in supervising their children's posture at home.

The personality and enthusiasm of the therapist must overcome these obstacles and inspire the patient, so that he wants to improve. This requires not only considerable personality, understanding and enthusiasm, but the ability to change routine quickly when boredom threatens.

Suggested Training Scheme

The basis of the postural training system described in this chapter consists of teaching the patient to adopt the correct posture in a number of different starting positions (which are graded progressively), and then training him to maintain a sound posture under all conditions of balance and during the ordinary movements of life. Mobility, strengthening, relaxation and balance exercises are also used.

When patients are taught as a group—and time and space allow it—informal activities and games are used throughout the training period to break up the more formal techniques. The activities and games help to provide generalized exercise, and are useful in increasing the respiratory excursions.

Two specimen postural training tables for children are given in chapter 7, p. 53.

SECTION 2: TEACHING GOOD POSTURE

(a) IN THE TREATMENT OF SPINAL DEFECTS*

Preliminary Approach

The patient is told something of his postural defects, and what is meant by good posture. As it is frequently necessary to teach some adjustment of the pelvis he is given some elementary instruction in the mechanics of pelvic and spinal movements, so that he understands the principles of the exercise treatment. A jointed cardboard model can be used with considerable success, especially when dealing with children. It is important that the explanation should be simple.

The Basis of the Training

The patient is first taught to correct his posture with the body in the horizontal position, so that the influence of gravity is eliminated. He progresses to postural correction in standing by a series of starting positions (p. 31), which gradually accustom him to controlling a greater number of joints in the vertical position.

Progression from one starting position to another is not allowed until the patient can maintain a correct posture in the easier position without undue effort. Generally, some weeks or months of training are required before the patient's normal standing posture is considered satisfactory.

Self-practice and self-correction. The success of the training depends largely on whether or not the patient can be persuaded to practise the training techniques on his own, and—what is extremely important—to try and hold himself correctly during the ordinary movements of life. For this reason it is essential that he should be shown how to carry out certain basic postural corrections in sitting and standing from the time the training is instituted. No serious attempt should be made, however, to re-educate his posture *completely* in these positions until he has progressed to them normally through the preliminary training positions.

* For convenience of description the treatment of postural defects of the spine and feet has been considered separately in Sections 2 and 3 of this chapter. In practice, however, it is unusual for one part of the body alone to be involved, and postural correction of the body as a whole is generally instituted. For Treatment of Postural "Flat Foot" *see* p. 34.

For example, the child with a lumbar lordosis and round shoulders, who spends much of his time at school in the sitting position, should be shown how to sit, write and work at his desk with the spine and scapulae held in a good position; this entails teaching him to move the trunk forward and backward at the hip joints without flexing the spine and rounding the shoulders. Similarly, he should be trained to maintain the correct position of the pelvis and scapulae when standing and when making common-place movements like sitting down and getting up from a chair. It is essential that the child should learn to achieve these corrections without holding himself in a stiff, unnatural manner.

Practical Considerations

Individual and group training. Individual training is necessary at first; later, when the postural training techniques are thoroughly understood, group instruction can be given (p. 53). Male and female patients should be treated separately; this applies particularly to children over the age of ten.

Clothing. Suitable clothing should be worn for the training. Male patients wear shorts or swimming trunks; female patients wear shorts or gym knickers and some form of chest covering which leaves the back as bare as possible. Gym shoes are generally worn.

A firm mattress or thick mat is used for all the lying positions.

Initial Training Techniques

The postural training techniques are started from crook lying (Fig. 11). The position has the advantage of discouraging any tendency on the part of the patient to hollow the lumbar spine.

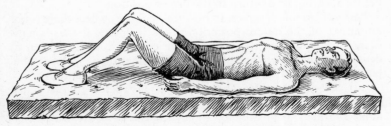

FIG. 11. Postural training. The first starting position: *crook lying*.

(i) *Gluteal contractions.* The patient is instructed in the technique of contracting the gluteal muscles in an isometric manner.

The extensor muscles of the hip joints, particularly the glutei, are used to decrease the pelvic inclination; the abdominal muscles, especially the recti, work in association with them in the performance of this function.

Conscious control of the gluteal muscles is extremely important. Because of the associated action of the abdominals with the glutei it is not necessary to teach abdominal contractions.

(ii) *Pelvic tilting.* Forward and backward tilting of the pelvis is next practised. The patient is then given instruction in the way in which he should adjust his pelvis if there is any deviation from the "normal" antero-posterior inclination.

Increased pelvic inclination. If the pelvic inclination is increased and the "normal" lumbar curve exaggerated (Lumbar lordosis, Fig. 2, p. 9, or Sway back, Fig. 3, p. 9), the patient is instructed to tilt the pelvis backward to the required degree, and maintain it in this position for a few moments before allowing it to return to its former position. When practising this technique in any of the positions where the spine rests against something firm, such as a mattress or wall, the patient generally finds it helpful to localize the correction by tilting the pelvis backward until the lumbar spine is pressed against the support. This exaggerated correction must only be used as an introductory measure, because it flattens the lumbar spine in an abnormal manner.

Decreased pelvic inclination. When the pelvic inclination is decreased and is associated with a flattening of the "normal" lumbar concavity (Flat back, Fig. 4, p. 10, and Round back, Fig. 5, p. 10), the patient is instructed to tilt the pelvis forward to the required degree and maintain it in this position for a few moments before allowing it to return to its former position.

Postural lateral curvature. In postural scoliosis, where there is no alteration of the antero-posterior pelvic inclination, the patient is instructed to keep the pelvis in the correct position. When a deviation from the "normal" pelvic inclination is present the patient is taught to correct this in the manner described above.

(iii) *Sub-costal angle.* The patient is instructed to place his hands on the sides of the lower thorax and open the sub-costal angle as widely as possible by expanding the lower ribs sideways. It is easier if the backs of the fingers rest on the sides of the thorax, with the metacarpo-phalangeal joints flexed, than if the palms of the hands are used.

The patient should open the sub-costal angle, hold it in position for a few moments, and then allow it to return to its former position. As the training continues he should endeavour to hold the angle open and allow the ribs to move normally during respiration.

(iv) *Thoracic spine.* The thoracic spine will be straightened automatically to a certain extent during the opening of the sub-costal angle, probably through the fixator action of the erector spinae. Further correction of the thoracic spine is difficult in crook lying, although it may be achieved by localized extension in the starting positions where the spine is held erect.

(v) *Scapulae and arms.* The shoulder joints are rotated laterally until the olecranon processes face backward; the radio-ulnar joints are then rotated medially so that the knuckles face outward. The fingers are loosely flexed.

Lateral rotation of the shoulder joints automatically places the scapulae in a good position because of the associated fixator action of the rhomboid muscles and the middle fibres of the trapezius. Direct correction of the scapulae is therefore generally unnecessary. If some correction is thought desirable it is better to instruct the patient to hold the scapulae "down" rather than "back".

When the patient understands how to correct the position of the scapulae by laterally rotating the shoulder joints, he should practise maintaining the scapulae in the corrected position while allowing the lateral rotator muscles of the shoulder joints to relax. This technique helps him to maintain a good position of the shoulder girdle when using the arms in normal, everyday activities, such as writing and eating, and when sitting in a sound " relaxed" position with the hands resting on the thighs (p. 20).

(vi) *Cervical spine.* The patient is told to draw the head up towards the wall, if the crown of the head is facing it, and to attempt to press the back of the neck gently against the mattress or mat *without* making a double chin. He maintains the correct position for a few moments and then allows the muscles of the neck to relax. Throughout, the chin should be level.

It is better to follow this technique of correcting the position of the head and neck than to instruct the patient to "pull in the chin", as is sometimes done. "Pulling in the chin" generally results in a gross over-tension of the muscles which control the movement, particularly the sterno-mastoid group.

Combining the Localized Movements

When the patient thoroughly understands how to carry out these techniques properly, he is asked to *combine* them in the order indicated and to hold the new position for a few moments. In this way he acquires the sense of correct posture. The time of "holding" the new position is gradually increased until the patient can maintain it continuously for several minutes without difficulty.

It is essential that after each part of the body has been moved it is held in its new position while the next movement takes place. This is not easy, and there is a tendency for the patient to relinquish control over certain muscle groups while activating other groups. A common error of this type is made when correcting the position of the scapulae. In concentrating on the arm movements the patient allows the pelvis and lumbar spine to return to their original, faulty position.

Avoiding a strained posture. At first, because of the concentrated effort required, the new position is stiff and unnatural. As the patient becomes more proficient at controlling his muscles he must attempt to slacken off the tension until his posture becomes natural and unstrained.

Exercising while maintaining the Correct Posture in Crook Lying

To assist the patient in cultivating good posture in crook lying he is trained to carry out simple arm and leg exercises while holding the rest of the body in the correct position. At first he finds this difficult, and in concentrating on the exercises may allow some of the muscles maintaining the correct position to relax.

The criterion of success is the patient's ability to maintain the correct posture *without undue effort* while exercising the arms and legs. This requires considerable practice.

Arm and Leg Exercises

The arm and leg exercises are given separately at first. Later, when the patient can maintain the correct posture while moving the arms or the legs, the movements of the limbs are combined.

Arm exercises. Any basic arm movements may be performed.

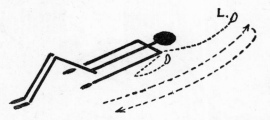

Fig. 12a. Cultivating good posture in crook lying by exercising each arm in turn while the rest of the body is held in the correct position. The left arm is bent to the fist bend position, and stretched sideways-upward, as shown; it is then returned to its original position by a reversal of the previous movements. The exercise is repeated with the right arm.

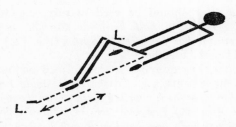

Fig. 12b. Cultivating good posture in crook lying by exercising each leg in turn. The left leg is stretched downward, the heel skimming the supporting surface; it is then returned to its original position by a reversal of the previous movement. The exercise is repeated with the right leg.

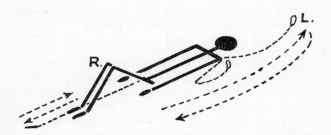

Fig. 12c. A combined arm and leg exercise based on the movements shown in Figs. 12a and 12b. The exercise is repeated with the right arm and left leg.

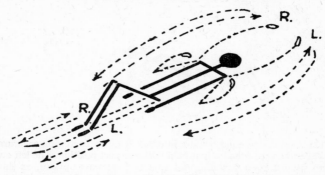

Fig. 12d. Another combined arm and leg exercise based on the movements shown in Figs. 12a and 12b. Both arms and legs are used at the same time.

Initially, the arms should be used in turn, e.g. *Crook lying; single Arm bending to half fist-bend position, and stretching sideways-upward to half lax-stretch position* (Fig. 12a). Later, both arms should be used together.

Leg exercises. Leg exercises are performed on the same lines as the arm movements, e.g. *Crook lying; single Leg stretching downward, skimming the supporting surface with the heel* (Fig. 12b).

Combined Arm and Leg exercises. Useful exercises include: (a) *Crook lying; single Arm bending to half fist-bend position, and stretching sideways-upward to half lax-stretch position, with opposite Leg stretching downward, the heel skimming the supporting surface* (Fig. 12c). (b) As previous exercise, but both arms are used together, first with one leg and then with the other. (c) *Crook lying; Arm bending to fist-bend position, and stretching sideways-upward to lax-stretch position, with Leg stretching downward, the heels skimming the supporting surface* (Fig. 12d).

Progressing by changing Starting Position

When the patient can control his posture successfully in crook lying while exercising the arms and legs, he should practice the postural corrections and exercises in the progressive starting positions given below. The leg exercises previously described must be modified slightly, to suit the different positions; they are omitted in kneel-sitting and kneeling, because of the difficulty of moving the lower limbs.

(*a*) Lying with the feet pressed against a wall (Fig. 13).
(*b*) Back-support-kneel-sitting (Fig. 14, p. 32).
(*c*) Kneel-sitting (Fig. 15, p. 32).
(*d*) Sitting (Fig. 9, p. 19).
(*e*) Kneeling (Fig. 16, p. 33).
(*f*) Back-lean-standing (Fig. 17, p. 33).
(*g*) Standing (Fig. 8, p. 18).

N.B. It cannot be stressed too strongly that the patient must not be allowed to progress from a starting position unless his ability to maintain a good posture in that position is of the standard suggested in the previous section, i.e. he can maintain the correct posture without undue effort while exercising the arms and legs.

(*a*) *Lying with the feet pressed against a wall* (Fig. 13). In this position postural training is applied to the body as a whole, as the lower limbs can be used in conjunction with the other parts.

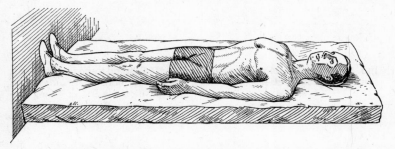

Fig. 13. Postural training. The second starting position: *lying with the feet pressed against a wall.*

The patient's feet project just beyond the end of the supporting mattress or mat, with the soles in contact with the wall, so that the ankle joints are dorsiflexed to 90°. The feet are held slightly apart—a gap of about two to three finger-breadths between the first metatarsal heads is a reasonable distance—with the toes and patellae pointing directly upward (Fig. 13).

The patient is instructed to press the feet gently against the wall without plantar-flexing the ankle joints. This produces an associated contraction of the extensor muscles of the knee and hip joints, as in standing. He is then told to maintain the foot pressure and to correct the rest of the body in the manner previously described under Initial Training Techniques (pp. 25–28). In this way the

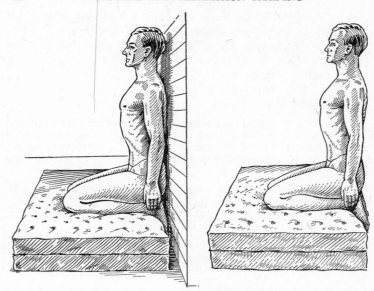

FIG. 14. Postural training. The third starting position: *back-support-kneel-sitting*.

FIG. 15. Postural training. The fourth starting position: *kneel-sitting*. The fifth position consists of sitting (*see* Fig. 9, p. 19).

patient acquires the sense of a good standing posture while in the lying position.

It should be noted that it is more difficult for the patient to correct a lumbar lordosis in lying than in crook lying, because the position tends to exaggerate the lumbar hollow.

Prone lying with the feet pressed against a wall is sometimes advocated as a progression on the lying position. Prone lying is not satisfactory in postural training because it is extremely difficult to achieve a good posture of the head and neck. For this reason it has not been included here.

(*b*) *Back-support-kneel-sitting* (Fig. 14). This position serves as an introductory to sitting and standing. The patient takes up the position on a pile of two or three mattresses as shown in Fig. 14, so that his feet are unsupported. The spine should be in contact with a wall or similar support, such as one of the upright posts

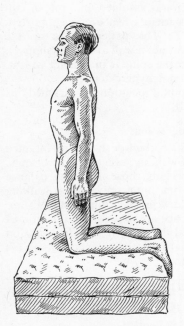

Fig. 16. Postural training. The sixth starting position: *kneeling*.

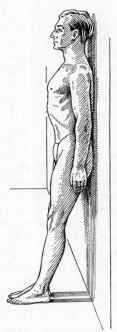

Fig. 17. Postural training. The seventh starting position: *back-lean-standing*. It is used as an introductory position to standing.

of the wall-bars. This helps the patient to isolate the spinal movements during the postural correction.

(*c*) *Kneel-sitting* (Fig. 15). The position is the same as the previous one, but the trunk is not held in contact with any supporting surface.

(*d*) *Sitting*. The patient assumes the correct sitting position on a chair or gymnasium stool,* as described on p. 19. If a gymnasium stool is used it should be arranged against a wall, so that the patient's trunk is supported. Later, the patient should practise sitting on the stool without support for the trunk.

---

* A wooden stool with a wide top which enables the patient to sit with the whole of the thighs supported, a right angle at the hip, knee and ankle joints, and the soles of the feet resting on the floor. *See* Fig. 57, p. 61.

(e) *Kneeling* (Fig. 16). The position is assumed on a pile of two or three mattresses, so that the patient's feet are unsupported.

(f) *Back-lean-standing* (Fig. 17). The patient takes up the position with his heels slightly in front of a wall or similar support, such as a wall-bar upright, so that the spine is in contact with it. The knee joints are extended but not hyperextended.

(g) *Standing*. The correct standing position is assumed, as described on p. 17 (*see* Fig. 8, p. 18).

Further Progressions

Walking and balance training. The correct posture is maintained while the patient practises normal walking, everyday movements, and simple balance exercises, especially those involving balance walking (*see* chapter 5, p. 39). When practising normal walking and everyday movements he should wear his ordinary shoes.

Points to stress in walking practice are: (a) correct position of the arms and hands as they swing at the sides (p. 18), (b) extension of the forward knee joint, (c) good heel-and-toe action, and (d) correct weight distribution on the foot.

SECTION 3: TEACHING GOOD POSTURE

(b) IN THE TREATMENT OF POSTURAL PES VALGUS*
(Postural " Flat Foot ")

Preliminary Approach

The nature of the foot defect should be explained to the patient in a simple manner. He should be shown clearly how the faulty position of the feet can be corrected by laterally rotating the hip joints to the required degree in standing.

Practical Considerations

Individual and group training. Individual training is necessary at first; later, group instruction can be given (p. 53). Male and female patients are generally treated separately, because in practice the training is rarely required for the foot defect alone but for the body as a whole.

* For convenience of description the treatment of postural defects of the spine and feet have been considered separately in Sections 2 and 3 of this chapter. In practice, however, it is unusual for one part of the body alone to be involved (*see* p. 7), and postural correction for the body as a whole is generally instituted.

Clothing. Suitable clothing should be worn for the training, as indicated on p. 25. At the beginning of the training the patient should be bare-footed. Later, when he can control the position of his feet and hip joints without difficulty, he may wear shoes during the training sessions.

Initial Training Technique

The initial corrective technique is best carried out from reach grasp standing, the wall-bars or a chair back being used (Fig. 18). The patient is instructed to rotate the hip joints laterally in a controlled manner, while keeping the feet firmly on the floor. The

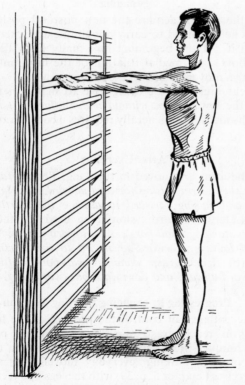

FIG. 18. Correction of postural pes valgue (postural "flat foot") from *reach grasp standing*. A chair back can be used instead of the wall-bars.

hip movement is continued until the valgus position of the feet has been corrected. The patient is then told to maintain the new posture of the legs for a few moments before allowing the limbs to return to their former position.

During the lateral rotation of the hips the patient is instructed to keep the toes pressed down straight against the floor or the shoe surface (p. 17), particularly the great toe. This counteracts the tendency for him to rock over on to the outer borders of the feet as he rotates the hip joints. The patient is also reminded to keep the knees extended.

Exercising while maintaining the Correct Posture in Reach Grasp Standing

To help the patient acquire the new postural position of the lower limbs he is trained to carry out simple arm exercises while maintaining it. At the beginning he usually finds this difficult, and may allow some medial rotation of the hip joints to occur during the arm movements.

The patient must aim at being able to maintain the correct posture of the lower limbs *without undue effort or tension* while exercising the arms. This generally requires a considerable amount of practice.

Arm Exercises

At first the arms are moved in turn, e.g. *Reach grasp standing (wall-bars); single Arm raising forward-upward, lowering sideways-downward, and raising forward to assume the starting position* (Fig. 19). Later, both arms should be used together, e.g. (a) *Reach grasp standing (wall-bars); Arm lowering, raising sideways-upward and lowering forward-downward to the starting position* (Fig. 20), (b) *Reach grasp standing (wall-bars); alternate Arm raising forward-upward and downward-backward* (Fig. 21).

Progressing by changing Starting Position

When the patient can control the posture of the lower limbs successfully in reach grasp standing, he should practise the training techniques in the correct standing position (p. 17). He must also practise walking, everyday movements, and simple balance exercises (chapter 5, p. 39) with the legs and feet corrected.

In walking the patient keeps the patellae facing directly forward, and holds the feet corrected when they are off the ground by

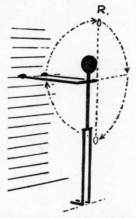

FIG. 19. Acquiring the new postural position of the legs by "holding" them correctly while exercising the arms. The reach grasp position can be taken at a chair back if wall-bars are not available. The right arm is raised forward-upward, lowered sideways-downward, and raised forward to grasp the wall-bar again. The exercise is repeated with the left arm.

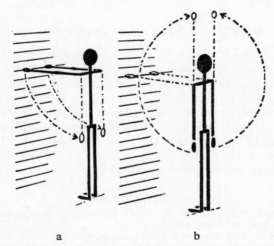

a   b

FIG. 20. Maintaining the new postural position of the legs while exercising the arms. From the reach grasp position the arms are lowered to the sides; they are then raised sideways-upward to the stretch position above the head; finally, they are lowered forward to grasp the bar again.

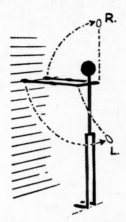

Fig. 21. Another arm exercise which is used while the legs are held in the correct position. From the reach grasp position each arm is raised alternately forward-upward and downward-backward.

adjusting the balance of the tibialis posterior and peroneus longus muscles.[2]

SECTION 4: TEACHING GOOD POSTURE

(c) In the Treatment of Genu Valgum and Genu Varum

Genu valgum or knock-knees. Postural training is not indicated in the treatment of knock-knees unless they are associated with a general faulty posture (p. 15). The training techniques described in the two previous sections are then employed (pp. 24 and 34).

Genu varum or bow legs. Postural training is used only in the treatment of apparent bow legs caused by faulty posture (p. 15). Training to correct the medial rotation of the legs is given as described in the previous section (p. 34).

REFERENCES

1. Wiles, P. and Sweetnam, R. (1965), *Essentials of Orthopaedics*, 4th ed., p. 34. London: J. and A. Churchill Ltd.
2. Wiles, P. and Sweetnam, R. (1965), *ibid*, p. 34.

Chapter 5

BALANCE EXERCISES

Balance exercises, especially those involving balance walking, are of considerable value in postural training, inasmuch as they give the patient excellent practice in maintaining and controlling his posture while the body is moving in a highly co-ordinated manner under varying conditions of balance. They also have the advantage of giving poise and grace to the carriage.

A useful series of balance exercises is given here, together with a brief description of balance walking techniques. The exercises have been arranged progressively in three main groups. They are performed with the patient either barefooted or wearing gym shoes.

Basic Exercises
Grade 1

1. Standing with back towards wall or wall-bars; single Knee raising. Each leg is raised, in turn, until there is a right angle at hip and knee, with the ankle joint plantar-flexed. The position is held for a moment or two; the leg is then lowered to its original place.
2. Standing with back towards wall or wall-bars; single Knee raising with Arm raising sideways. As above, but during the knee raising the arms are raised sideways to the horizontal position, palms facing downwards.
3. Standing with back towards wall or wall-bars; single Knee raising, Leg stretching forward to 45°, and slow lowering.
4. Balance walking forward and backward along a straight line. *See* Balance walking technique, p. 43.
5. Toe balance walking sideways along a straight line. *See* Balance walking technique, p. 44.

Grade 2

1. Balance walking forward and backward with Knee raising.
2. Balance walking forward and backward with opposite Knee and Arm raising. Fig. 22.
3. No progression.
4. Balance half standing* (balance bench rib); balance walking forward and backward.

* Standing on one foot on balance bench rib or beam, with the other leg hanging free, as shown in Fig. 33, p. 45.

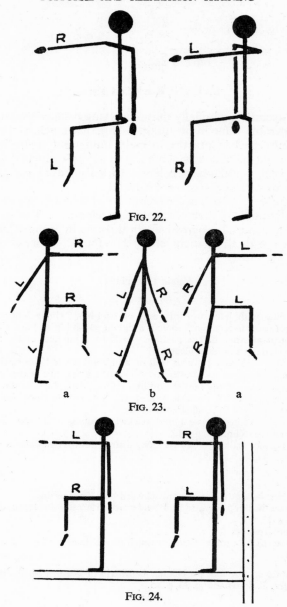

FIG. 22.

a   b   a

FIG. 23.

FIG. 24.

5. Across balance standing* (balance bench rib); balance walking sideways with heels kept low to let the feet grip the rib.

Intermediate Exercises
Grade 1

1. Balance half standing† (balance bench rib or beam); balance walking forward and backward with Knee raising.

1a. Balance walking forward with Knee and Arm raising of the same side, and opposite Arm raising backward. Fig. 23.

2. Balance half standing (balance bench rib or beam); balance walking forward and backward with opposite Knee and Arm raising. Fig. 24.

3. No progression.

4. Balance half standing (balance bench rib: sloping bench); balance walking forward and backward. Fig. 25.

5. Across balance standing* (beam); balance walking sideways with heels kept low to let the feet grip the beam.

Grade 2

1. No progression.

1a. Balance half standing† (balance bench rib or beam); balance walking forward with Knee and Arm raising of the same side, and opposite Arm raising backward. Fig. 23 shows the exercise performed without apparatus.

2-3. No progressions.

4. Balance half standing (balance bench rib: bench arranged as see-saw); balance walking forward and backward. *See* Fig. 51, p. 58.

5. No progression.

6. Balance half standing (balance bench rib or beam); toe balance walking forward to 3 counts, followed by Knee full bending and stretching to 6 counts. Fig. 26.

Advanced Exercises
Grade 1

1-3. No progressions.

4. Balance half standing† (balance bench rib or beam); balance walking forward, bouncing a ball from side to side of bench or beam. Fig. 27.

4a. Balance half standing (balance bench rib or beam); balance walking forward, throwing a ball from hand to hand. Fig. 28.

5. No progression.

6. Balance half standing (balance bench rib or beam); toe balance walking forward, at given count assuming lax stoop full knee bend position with knees forward. Fig. 29.

* Standing on balance bench rib or beam, with feet at right angles to rib or beam, weight taken on balls of feet. *See* Fig. 32, p. 45.

† Standing on one foot on balance bench rib or beam, with the other leg hanging free, as shown in Fig. 33, p. 45.

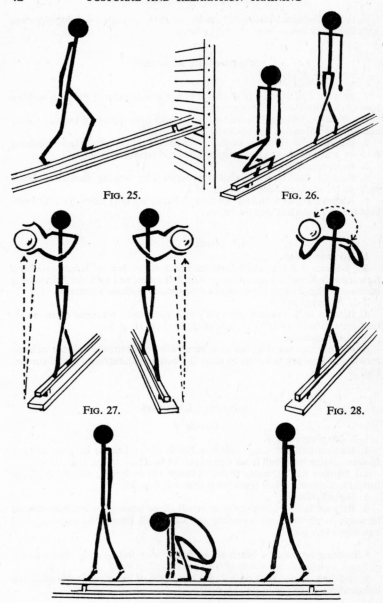

FIG. 25.

FIG. 26.

FIG. 27.

FIG. 28.

FIG. 29.

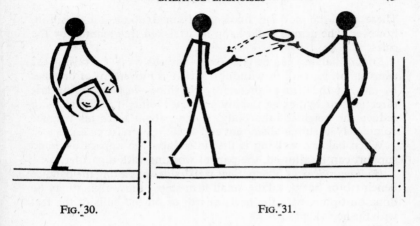

FIG. 30.   FIG. 31.

Grade 2

1–3. No progressions.

4. Balance half standing* (beam); balance walking forward with Knee raising, passing a ball under raised knee. Fig. 30.

4a. Balance half standing (beam: partners at opposite ends, facing each other); balance walking forward and backward, throwing a quoit to each other. Fig. 31.

5–6. No progressions.

TECHNIQUE OF BALANCE WALKING ON BALANCE
BENCH RIB OR BEAM

Walking forward and backward. The patient places the free foot in front of the other one, so that the heels are slightly more than a foot-length apart. The body weight is transferred to it, and then the other leg is placed in front of it, as previously described. This is repeated until the patient reaches the end of the apparatus. He should then walk backward, the same procedure being repeated, with the exception that the leading leg is carried behind the trunk. As in all balance walking the forefoot is put down first on the supporting surface, and then the heel.

To acquire a good balancing technique the patient should learn to place the feet accurately without having to look down. He should hold the trunk straight and the head erect, with the eyes fixed on some point directly in front and at their own level.

* Standing on one foot on balance bench rib or beam, with the other leg hanging free, as shown in Fig. 33, p. 45.

There must be nothing fixed or strained about the position, however. The arms should hang in a relaxed free manner by the sides.

Loss of balance can be restored in various ways: by raising the arms sideways, with or without a sideways movement of one leg; by moving the trunk—preferably the hips—in the appropriate direction; or by flexing the hip and knee joints quickly, so as to reduce the height of the body. If the patient loses his balance completely he should dismount and start the exercise again.

When balance walking is first introduced on apparatus, hand support can be allowed, the patient working with a partner.

Walking sideways. The patient walks sideways along the balance bench rib or beam, taking small firm steps; the walking may be done on tiptoe, with the heels raised, or on the balls of the feet with the heels kept low.

The balance technique is the same as that described for balance walking forward and backward, but the arms are generally held loosely forward to maintain balance. When the walking is introduced hand support can be allowed, the patient working with his partner. Fig. 32.

Turning through 90° or 180° from balance standing. The patient raises the heels slightly, and then turns either slowly or quickly on the balls of the feet to the side of the rear leg. He may find it helpful to raise the arms sideways as he turns, and use them to assist his balance.

TECHNIQUE OF MOUNTING APPARATUS

Balance bench rib. The patient stands sideways on to the balance bench, which is arranged with the rib uppermost. He places the foot of the near leg on the rib and steps up, so as to assume a half standing position with the foot of the other leg hanging down by the side of the rib. Fig. 33.

Patients frequently mount the rib from one end. This can be dangerous, because after one foot has been placed on the end of the rib, the other foot is often put down on the projecting base piece, which may cause the bench to tip sideways.

Beam arranged up to knee height. The patient mounts as previously described.

Beam arranged between knee and hip height. The patient faces the beam and grasps it with both hands, fingers forward. He then places the inner border of one foot on the beam, with the knee

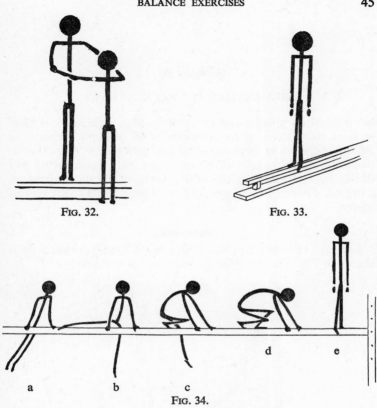

FIG. 32.

FIG. 33.

a   b   c   d   e

FIG. 34.

kept straight, and mounts it in the manner demonstrated in Fig. 34.

DISMOUNTING FROM APPARATUS

From the beam. Normally the patient dismounts by a reversal of the mounting technique. If he needs to dismount quickly during a balance exercise, however, the method to be followed depends on the height of the beam. Up to hip height he generally jumps sideways; above this height he stoops down quickly, grasps the beam and jumps sideways.

From the balance bench rib. The patient dismounts by a reversal of the mounting technique. If a quick descent is needed he usually jumps sideways.

Chapter 6

PREVENTION OF BACK STRAIN

No manual on posture and postural training would be complete without reference to practical methods of avoiding ligamentous strains of the spine. Such strains occur with almost monotonous regularity among adults of all ages, not only during work but during the ordinary activities of life. Many of the strains produce a degree of backache and pain out of all proportion to the type of injury.

Housework

Lifting. The wrong way of lifting a heavy load from the floor is shown in Fig. 35. The spine is flexed and vulnerable.

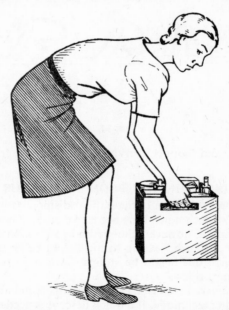

FIG. 35. Wrong way of lifting: spine flexed and vulnerable.

46

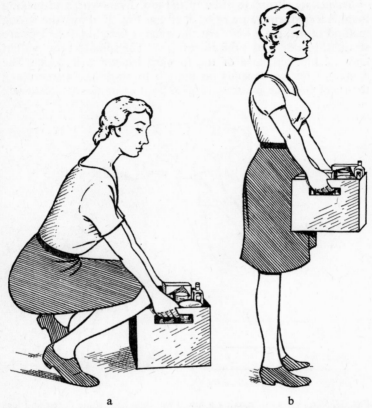

a   b

FIG. 36. Right way of lifting for the housewife: hips and knees well flexed and spine straight with lumbar region slightly hollowed. Most housewives prefer this lifting position to the one used by heavy manual workers where the knees are parted widely, as shown in Fig. 39b, p. 51.

The right way of lifting is shown in Fig. 36. The knees and hips are flexed and the back kept slightly hollow. Professional weight-lifters always adopt the hollow position of the back when lifting because they have found from experience that it prevents strain.

The same method of lifting should be used by a mother when picking up a child from the floor. The knees are then parted. *See* Fig. 39b, p. 51.

Bedmaking. Beds are often of the low divan type, and making them is a frequent cause of back strain. Fig. 37 shows the wrong method of making a low bed: the spine is flexed and the legs are straight. Fig. 38 shows the correct way. The spine is kept straight and the hip and knee of the forward leg are well flexed. The degree of flexion depends on the job to be done. In smoothing the sheet over the mattress (Fig. 38), for example, the housewife

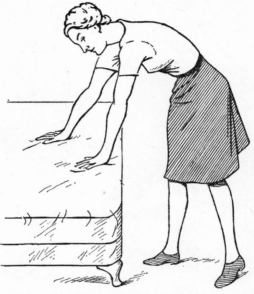

FIG. 37. Wrong way of making a low divan-type bed: spine flexed and legs straight.

does not flex at the hip and knee as much as when tucking in the bedclothes.

Avoiding strain in standing. Whenever possible the housewife should avoid too much standing while working in the kitchen, and there are many jobs she can do in sitting, even if this goes against the grain. A high stool is a help in this connection. She should also arrange kitchen utensils, and equipment in constant use, at levels which do not necessitate bending.

Some forms of work cannot be managed satisfactorily in sitting, and necessitate fairly long periods of standing. The housewife can protect her feet from too much strain by standing on the outer borders (with the feet fully inverted) for *short* periods.

Carrying. When carrying a heavy tray upstairs the housewife should lean slightly forward from the hips, keeping the tray close to her body; the elbows should be kept at the sides. When she is out shopping with a full and heavy basket she should endeavour to keep the body as erect as possible against the weight, and change the basket fairly frequently from one hand to the other.

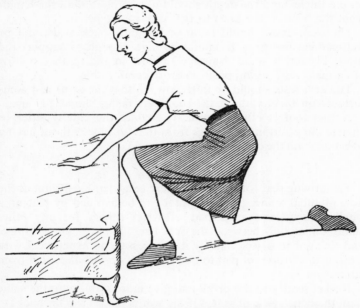

FIG. 38. Right way of making a low bed: spine straight and hip and knee of forward leg well flexed.

Pushing. In pushing a heavy piece of furniture the housewife should keep her knees slightly flexed, and the spine upright. She should stand near to the object to be moved. One foot should be close to it, and the other a pace or so behind; this allows her to obtain the required leverage.

Sitting and the Elderly

Most old people spend a considerable amount of their time sitting in an armchair. Often the chair is of the deep, soft type—

the seat is too low, it tends to "give" too much, and its depth from front to back is too great. These factors allow the spine to assume a slumped, flexed posture, with the head poked forward. The head and neck position is made worse if TV is watched for several hours each day.

Preferably, the armchair should be of the winged variety, with a fairly firm, but not hard, seat. The seat should be high enough to allow the feet to rest easily on the floor without undue pressure on the thighs, and the depth should not be more than the length from the back of the knee to the back of the pelvis.

The chair back should be angled slightly backwards, and be well-padded but firm. It should be high enough to support the head. Placing a small "sausage" pillow in the lumbar hollow often makes the sitting position more comfortable.

The arm rests should be fairly low, so that the arms rest comfortably on them without the shoulders being "hunched" up.

A footstool is often helpful. It enables the elderly sitter to change the position of the legs from time to time without having to get up from the chair.

Driving

The driving seats of some cars cause considerable flexion of the dorso-lumbar spine. Lumbar strain can be avoided by placing a small rectangular-shaped pad of foam rubber (or any other suitable material) between the seat back and the lumbar spine, and tieing it in place. Usually it is necessary to experiment with various thicknesses of pad to obtain both comfort and relief from strain.

Bucket seats grip the pelvis and give more stability to the spine than the bench type of seat. "If the seat is placed too far back, so that the knees are extended, the use of the foot pedals will cause a constant movement of the pelvic ring at its articulation with the spine at the lumbo-sacral joint, and stretching of the sacro-iliac ligaments. Sacro-iliac strain can be avoided by moving the seat forward to a position where the driver's knees are flexed when the pedals are fully depressed.

"The bench seat is orthopaedically undesirable, because it gives no point of fixation except at the back, and relies on friction to stop the buttocks from sliding from side to side, because only feet and hands are tethered. Use of seat belts affords additional fixation." [1]

Gardening

Digging. When lifting a spadeful of earth the gardener should flex at the knees and hips, keeping the spine as straight as possible. If he has a considerable amount of digging to do he should learn to handle the spade with a right and left-hand action, but this requires time and patience.

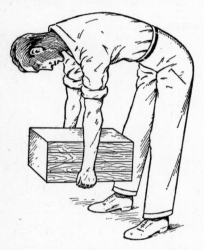 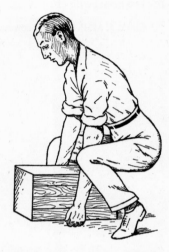

FIG. 39a. Wrong way of lifting for heavy manual workers: knees straight and spine flexed.	FIG. 39b. Right way of lifting: hips and knees well flexed, spine straight with lumbar region hollowed.

Weeding from standing is a constant source of back strain because it combines flexion and rotation. It is far better to kneel on a foam rubber pad, with a piece of polythene sheeting placed under it if the ground is damp. Bedding out of plants and bulb planting can also be done from kneeling.

In using lawn mowers—particularly the manual types—the spine must be kept straight and not allowed to "crouch" over the handles.

Long-handled tools, such as the bedding fork and lawn-edging shears, should be used whenever possible, as they necessitate the minimum of spinal flexion.

Heavy Manual Work

The methods previously described for preventing back strain apply equally to workers in heavy industry, although they may be far more difficult to apply. Fig. 39b shows the right method of lifting a heavy load from the ground, and Fig. 39a the wrong way. The correct technique is the same basically as that recommended for the housewife (Fig. 36a), but the knees are kept well apart.

[1] Clark, J. M. P. Personal communication.

Chapter 7

POSTURAL TRAINING TABLES FOR CHILDREN

Indications for Use

In the treatment of children, aged ten to fifteen, who are suffering from postural defects of the spine and feet (pp. 8–15). The tables may also be used in cases where the defects are of an isolated nature, e.g. postural lateral curvature unassociated with valgus feet. The exercises and training techniques which are not required are then omitted from the tables.

Group Instruction

The tables have been designed for small groups of patients, six to eight at the most. When the postural training techniques are first introduced each patient is given individual instruction; later, when the techniques are thoroughly understood, the patients either practise on their own, the instructor giving individual coaching as required, or work as a class. It is probable that certain patients will be at different stages of postural progress; some may therefore practise the techniques in one starting position, others in another.

The exercises which are used to supplement the postural training techniques are usually carried out on class lines.

Time Required

Approximately forty-five to sixty minutes. Each table can be shortened by combining some of the exercises and omitting the team game and some of the informal activities.

As the patients' posture improves certain of the exercises may be omitted, e.g. the relaxation exercises and some of the mobility and strengthening exercises.

Clothing

Suitable clothing should be worn for the training, as described on p. 25.

TABLE 1

For use when Gymnastic Apparatus is Available

1. **Introductory activity:**	Here; There; Where (*see* p. 62, Games Supplement).
2. ***Mobility exercises:**	(*a*) Stride standing; Trunk bending from side to side (Fig. 40).
Spine	(*b*) Side lying; Trunk bending forward with high Knee raising, followed by Trunk and Leg stretching backward, and return to starting position (Fig. 41).
	(*c*) Prone kneeling; Trunk turning with single Arm swinging sideways-upward and rhythmical pressing to 3 counts (Fig. 42).
Shoulder girdles	(*d*) Sitting; Shoulder rolling with emphasis on the backward movements (Fig. 43).
Shoulder joints	(*e*) Fist bend crook lying; alternate Arm stretching sideways-upward (Fig. 44).
Feet	(*f*) Sitting (one ankle crossed over the opposite knee); single Foot circling continuously to a given count.
3. **Informal activity:**	Chinese Boxing (*see* p. 63, Games Supplement).
4. **Postural Training Techniques:**	*Session* 1. (10 minutes approximately.) Spine and Shoulder girdles (*see* pp. 25–34). Feet (*see* pp. 34–36).
5. **Minor game:**	Balls Passing (*see* p. 66, Games Supplement).
6. **General strengthening exercises:**	(*a*) Fixed prone lying; Trunk bending backward with Arm turning outward (Fig. 45, p. 56).
Spine	(*b*) Stretch grasp back toward standing (wall bars); high Knee raising (Fig. 46, p. 56).
	(*c*) Fixed side lying (one leg in front of the other) Trunk bending sideways (Fig. 47, p. 56).
	(*d*) Yard (palms backward) half crook half vertical leg lift lying; Leg lowering sideways (Fig. 48, p. 57).
Retractors of scapulae	(*e*) Sitting; Shoulder bracing with Arm turning outward (Fig. 49, p. 57).
Lateral rotators of hips	(*f*) Prone lying; single Leg raising backward with turning outward (Fig. 50, p. 57).
Invertors of feet	(*g*) Sitting: Foot shortening (raising of medial longitudinal arches with flexion of metatarso-phalangeal joints, the toes being pressed down against the floor in their entire length).
7. **Informal activity:**	French Touch (*see* p. 63, Games Supplement).

* If mobility exercises are not required, rhythmical free standing "preparatory" exercises for the body as a whole may be given.

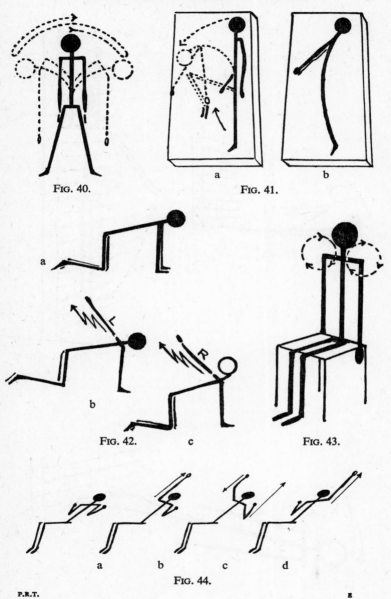

Fig. 40.

Fig. 41.

Fig. 42.

Fig. 43.

Fig. 44.

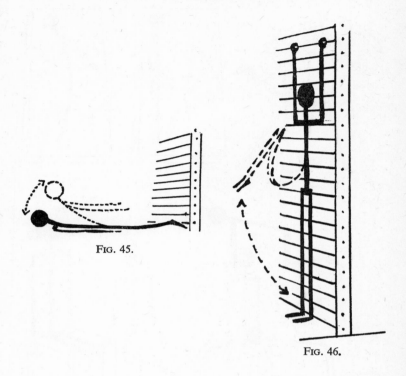

Fig. 45.

Fig. 46.

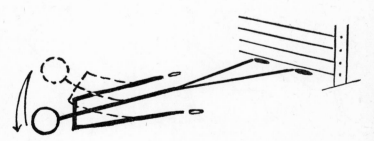

Fig. 47.

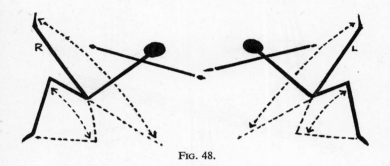

FIG. 48.

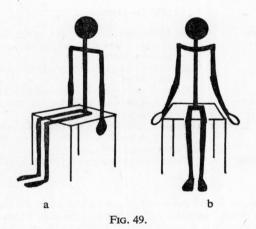

a   b

FIG. 49.

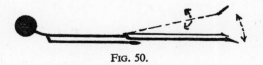

FIG. 50.

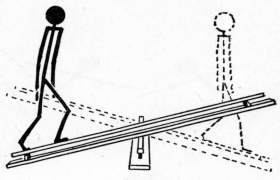

FIG. 51.

TABLE 1—*continued.*

8. Relaxation training:	(*a*) Lying; general relaxation (*see* p. 74). (*b*) Sitting; Shoulder shrugging and bracing, followed by relaxation. (*c*) Crook lying; Head pressing backward, and relaxation.
9. Balance exercises:	Balance half standing (balance bench rib: bench arranged as see-saw); balance walking forward and backward (Fig. 51).
10. Postural Training Techniques:	*Session* 2. (10 minutes approximately.) Spine and Shoulder Girdles (*see* pp. 25–34). Feet (*see* pp. 34–36).
11. Minor Team game:	Team Passing (*see* p. 67, Games Supplement).

N.B. When the patient can maintain a good posture in the lying position with the feet pressed against a wall (p. 31), three specific informal activities which help to cultivate a sound postural sense can be introduced into the table in addition to, or in place of, the informal activities suggested. A fourth specific activity may be introduced when the patient can maintain a good posture in standing (p. 17). The specific informal activities are described on p. 61, Games Supplement.

TABLE 2

For use when Gymnastic Apparatus is not available

1. **Introductory activity:**	One against Three (*see* p. 65, Games Supplement).
2. ***Mobility exercises:**	(*a*) Stride standing; Trunk bending sideways with rhythmical pressing to 3 counts.
Spine	(*b*) Side lying; Trunk bending forward with high Knee raising, followed by Trunk and Leg stretching backward, and return to starting position (*see* Fig. 41, p. 55).
	(*c*) Stride standing; Trunk turning from side to side with Arm swinging loosely at the sides.
Shoulder girdles	(*d*) Sitting; Shoulder bracing and rounding, with emphasis on bracing.
	(*e*) Sitting; Shoulder shrugging followed by strong Shoulder depression.
Shoulder joints	(*f*) Sitting or standing; Arm swinging forward and downward-sideways (Fig. 52, p. 60).
Feet	(*g*) Sitting (one ankle crossed over the opposite knee); single Foot circling continuously to a given count.
3. **Informal activity:**	Knee Boxing: (*see* p. 66. Games Supplement).
4. **Postural Training Techniques:**	*Session* 1. (10 minutes approximately). Spine and Shoulder Girdles (*see* pp. 25–34). Feet (*see* pp. 34–36).
5. **Minor game:**	Centre Circle Pass Ball (*see* p. 66, Games Supplement).
6. **General strengthening exercises:**	(*a*) Prone lying; Trunk bending backward with Arm turning outward and single Leg raising backward (Fig. 53).
Spine	(*b*) Lying; high Knee raising, followed by over-pressure with the hands, and upper Trunk bending forward (Fig. 54).
	(*c*) Low reach grasp standing (chair back); Hip updrawing (Fig. 55, p. 60).
	(*d*) Stride sitting (chair); Trunk turning with Arm moving loosely sideways in the direction of the turning to grasp the chair back (Fig. 56, p. 60).
Retractors of scapulae	(*e*) Yard (palms forward) crook lying; Shoulder bracing.
Lateral rotators of hips	(*f*) Prone lying; single Leg raising backward with turning outward (*see* Fig. 50, p. 57).
Invertors of feet	(*g*) Sitting; inner Border raising with Toe bending.

* If mobility exercises are not required, rhythmical free standing "preparatory" exercises for the body as a whole may be given.

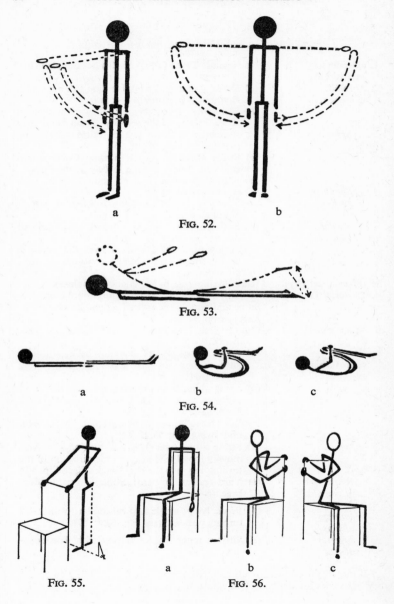

Fig. 52.

Fig. 53.

Fig. 54.

Fig. 55.

Fig. 56.

TABLE 2—*continued.*

7. **Informal activity:**	Touching opposite Ear and Nose (*see* p. 63, Games Supplement).
8. **Relaxation training:**	(*a*) Lying; general relaxation (*see* p. 74).
	(*b*) Sitting; Shoulder shrugging and bracing, followed by relaxation.
	(*c*) Crook lying; Head pressing backward, and relaxing.
9. **Balance exercises:**	Walking freely, attempt to kick the Hand held forward every 3rd step (opposite hand to leg). Variation: Toe walking.

10. **Postural Training Techniques:**   *Session 2.*   (10 minutes approximately.)
Spine and Shoulder Girdles (*see* pp. 25–34).
Feet (*see* pp. 34–36).

11. **Minor Team game:**	Team Passing (*see* p. 67, Games Supplement).

N.B. For introduction of specific informal activities *see* Note, p. 58.

GAMES SUPPLEMENT

The activities and games used in the previous tables are fully described in this section, together with some other activities and games which are useful in postural training.

1. SPECIFIC POSTURAL ACTIVITIES

Prone balancing. The patient lies across the top of a balance bench or gymnasium stool in the prone position, with the arms at the sides, so that the body is completely balanced (Fig. 57). He corrects his posture, with the help of his partner or the therapist, and endeavours to maintain it.

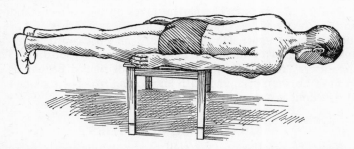

FIG. 57. *Prone balancing:* an informal activity which helps to cultivate a sound postural sense. The activity should not be used until the patient can maintain a good posture in the lying position with the feet pressed against a wall (p. 31).

Prone balancing with arm movements. As the previous activity, but simple arm movements are added, e.g. *single Arm bending to half fist-bend position, and stretching sideways-upward to half lax-stretch position* (*see* Fig. 12a, p. 29).

Prone balancing: passing bean bag over body. The patient lies across a gymnasium stool in the prone position with the arms to the sides, so that the body is completely balanced. A bean bag is placed on the floor a short distance in front of him (Fig. 58).

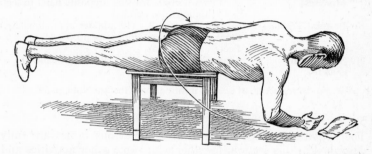

FIG. 58. A more difficult postural activity: *Prone balancing—passing bean bag over back.*

The patient corrects his posture with the help of his partner or the therapist. He then reaches down with one hand and attempts to pick up the bag, pass it over his back to the other hand, and return it to the floor (Fig. 58). Throughout, he must maintain the correct posture and his balance. This is extremely difficult.

Rocking the dummy. The patient takes up the correct standing position between two supporters, who face each other and are a short distance apart. He falls forward and backward from the ankle joints, with the body held in the correct posture. The supporters "receive" him with their hands placed behind or in front of his shoulders, and push him to and fro. The rocking can also be done in a sideways direction.

2. INFORMAL ACTIVITIES

Here; There; Where. One wall of the gymnasium represents *Here*; another wall—usually the opposite one—*There*; and the centre of the gymnasium represents *Where*.

The therapist gives brisk, rapid commands—e.g. "There!" . . . "Where!" . . . "Here!" . . . "Where!" . . . "There!" . . . "Here!" —and the players run to the areas indicated. The object is to tax the reactions of the players as much as possible by a quick change of command. A conversational type of approach by the therapist is very useful also: "If Here is There, Where can There be? . . . Surely not over Here! Of course, Where *can* be There, and Here can be Where, but who knows Where . . . There is? . . ." and so on.

Variation. The players carry out skip-jumping or some similar type of activity in the centre of the gymnasium on the command Where!

Chinese Boxing. The players face each other in pairs. They raise their arms forward-upward until they are almost fully elevated. Each player then grasps his partner's *left* wrist with his right hand. On the signal to start he attempts to touch his partner's forehead with his right hand, while the partner resists the attempt with his left arm. The players struggle against each other, pushing forward and backward. The therapist encourages them by suitable coaching.

On the command " Change!" the hand grasp is altered; each player holds his partner's right wrist with his left hand, and attempts to touch his forehead with the left hand in the manner previously described.

French touch. A player is selected by the therapist to be the tagger. On the signal to start he attempts to touch any one of the other players, who run in all directions in order to avoid him. The tagger may touch the players on any part of the body, but he should aim at touching some aspect of the lower limbs. When a player has been touched he becomes the tagger, while the previous tagger joins the other players. The new tagger must hold the area touched with one hand until he has succeeded in tagging a player himself.

Touching the opposite Ear and Nose. At the signal to begin each player attempts to touch (*a*) his right ear with his left hand while touching his nose with the other hand, and (*b*) his left ear with his right hand while touching his nose with the other hand. The touching is carried out continuously for a given number of times, e.g. 8–10. The first player to complete the full number of touches puts up his hand and is awarded a point.

Variation. The ear and nose touching is alternated with hand-clapping in front of the chest. For example, (a) Left hand on right ear and right hand on nose, (b) right hand on left ear and left hand on nose, (c) hand-clapping in front of chest four times, (d) repeat of (a) and (b), and (e) hand-clapping in front of chest four times.

Heading, Saving and Kicking an imaginary Football. The players are asked to mime the actions of heading, saving and kicking a football. The activity can be coached in two ways.

Method 1. The therapist indicates the direction in which the players should "head", "save" or "kick". The order of the movements should be varied, e.g. "Save it to the right! . . . Kick it to the left! . . . Head it forward! . . ."

Method 2. The therapist gives a running commentary on an imaginary soccer match, while the players mime the actions suggested. For example, "Ball's been kicked to the left . . . now it's been kicked forward! It's been headed to the right . . . the goalkeeper's brought off a wonderful save to the left! . . ."

In the Pond, On the Bank, In the Air, In the Trees. Certain positions are chosen to represent the various "situations" given here. For example, (a) In the Pond by lying, (b) On the Bank by lying with one or both legs abducted, (c) In the Air by lying with one leg raised to 45°, and (d) In the Trees by lying with the arms stretched forward. The therapist calls out the various "situations" and the players must immediately assume the appropriate positions. The order in which the "situations" are given must be varied as much as possible, e.g. "In the Air! . . . In the Trees! . . . On the Bank! . . . In the Air! . . . In the Air! . . . On the Bank!"

A conversational method of coaching can be used very successfully for this activity. For example, the therapist might say: "If I were in the Trees, I wouldn't be on the Bank or in the Pond, or in the Air. Of course, it would never do to fall in the Pond, would it? To get on the Bank might be very difficult, so I think I'd rather stay on the Bank, or in the Air, or even in the Trees— anywhere, in fact, but in the Pond . . ."

Do This, Do That. The therapist demonstrates a number of different movements to the players, using two commands only: *Do This!* and *Do That!* Movements demonstrated to the command "Do This!" must be performed by the players; those demonstrated to the command "Do That!" must be ignored. At the end of the activity the therapist should ascertain the number of players who were not "caught out"; a point is awarded to each successful player.

The activity can be coached in a conversational manner, the therapist demonstrating various movements as he talks. For example, he might say: "If I were to Do This, you would say that I was going to Do That, but of course to Do This isn't to Do That. It really is difficult, when to Do That I have to Do This, and sometimes I think it would be easier to just Do This, or Do That, or even to Do That again . . ."

One against Three. The players divide up into groups of four. Three of the players, holding each other's wrists firmly form a circle; the fourth player "marks" one of the players and stands on the opposite side of the circle to him. On the signal to start the fourth player attempts to tag the "marked" player, the rest of the players attempting to prevent him from doing so by turning and dodging without breaking their circle formation. When the player has been tagged the fourth man takes his place in the circle and the "marked" player now becomes the "tagger". The next player to be "marked" must be someone other than the fourth player who has just joined the circle.

Dodge and Mark. The players arrange themselves in pairs; one player is the runner, and the other the chaser. On the signal to start the runner tries to get away from the chaser by running, swerving and dodging. The chaser attempts to keep within touching distance of the runner, so that when the signal to stop is given he can touch him.

Poison. Three or more players, holding each other's wrists firmly, are grouped round a circle of about 4–5 feet in diameter. On the signal to start everyone pulls and pushes in an attempt to force another player into the circle. A point is awarded against any player who steps into the circle.

A variation of this activity is played with an object such as an Indian club or a medicine ball in the centre of the circle. Everyone attempts to force another player to touch the object.

Running, Jumping to touch object held by Leader, and over marked spaces. The therapist marks out, at suitable intervals, a number of squares on the floor. He then stands on a form which is placed at some distance from the squares and holds out a stick so that it is almost out of reach of the players. On the signal to start the players run round the gymnasium in file, jumping over the marked squares on the floor and jumping up to touch the stick as they pass under it.

Instead of using a form and a stick the therapist can stand on the wall-bars and hold out his arm for the players to touch.

Knee Boxing. The players stand facing each other in pairs. On the signal to start each player tries to touch his opponent on the knee with his open hand, at the same time attempting to prevent his own knees from being touched. The players must move about freely as in boxing.

3. MINOR GAMES (GROUP)

Balls passing. The players stand astride in circle formation. On the signal to start they pass two footballs round the circle, each player handling the balls in turn. At the beginning of the game one ball is passed slightly before the other. At suitable intervals the therapist commands "Change!" and the direction of the ball-passing is reversed. When a player receives both footballs at the same time a point is awarded against him.

Three footballs may be used if the circle formation is fairly large. If sufficient players are present two or more circles can be formed and the game may be made competitive.

Steps and Statues. The players stand facing a wall or a line. One player is chosen to be the statue; he stands facing the backs of the other players, and about 8 or 10 yards away from them. On the signal to start he endeavours to approach the players— without being detected in the act of moving forward—and touch one of them. The players may turn to look backward whenever they feel that the statue is moving, but must not leave the wall or line. If the statue is observed in "motion", he must return to his starting place; if he succeeds in touching one of the players without being detected, the "touched" player becomes the statue.

Centre-circle Pass Ball. The players all sit on stools and are arranged in circle formation, with one player (No. 1) in the centre. The players forming the circle face the centre player and are spaced well apart (Fig. 59). Players Nos. 1 and 2 each hold a football.

At the signal to start No. 2 passes the ball to No. 3, who passes it to No. 4, and so on, the ball moving continuously round the circle. After a brief pause No. 1 passes his football to No. 2, who returns it to him; he then passes the ball to No. 3, who returns it to him. He repeats this process with each player in turn, the

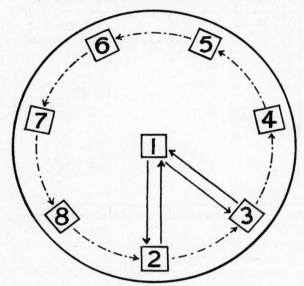

FIG. 59. Plan of Centre Circle Pass Ball.

passing being carried out in a continuous manner. When a player (e.g. No. 4) receives both footballs at the same time, he and No. 1 exchange places. On the signal to restart the game the direction of the ball-passing is changed. No. 4 passes to No. 3, and No. 3 passes to No. 2, and so on. From the centre of the circle, after a brief pause, No. 1 passes to No. 4, then to Nos. 3 and 2, and so on.

4. MINOR GAME (TEAM)

Team Passing. Apparatus: A football. *Formation:* The players divide up into two equal teams. No special formation is required, although it is best if the players start the game by being paired off in opposing couples as indicated in Fig. 60.

Method of play. The ball is put into play by the therapist bouncing it between two opposing players. The players of one team attempt to pass the ball among themselves, while the players of the other team try to intercept it and monopolize the passing. A set number of *consecutive* passes is the aim of each team, e.g. eight consecutive passes.

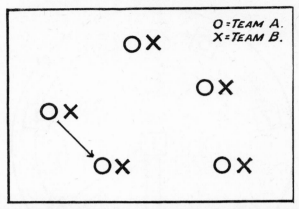

FIG. 60. Plan showing formation of players for *Team Passing*.

The game is usually played for about five minutes only, as it is extremely strenuous. Players must spread out throughout the game, as passes are more easily made among the outer players.

Rules: (*a*) Holding the ball for more than three seconds is not allowed.

        (*b*) Travelling more than two steps with the ball is not permitted.

        (*c*) No form of rough play is allowed.

        (*d*) If, after a pass has been made, the receiving player *immediately* returns the ball to the thrower, no further point is awarded.

        (*e*) If the ball is held by two opposing players at the same time, the therapist restarts the game.

Penalty: Free throw to opponents.

PART TWO: RELAXATION TRAINING

Chapter 8

INDICATIONS FOR RELAXATION TRAINING

Living muscles are said to be relaxed, or at rest, when they are relatively free from tension. Even in the relaxed state, however, they are never absolutely free from tension, because their basic physiological activity produces a degree of firmness.

Under certain circumstances abnormal muscular tension exists, and training in the art of relaxation is often prescribed to counteract its effects. The tension may be general in character due to mental anxiety or fear, as is apparent, for example, in psychosomatic tension states, or it may be of a more localized nature as a result of some alteration in the normal body mechanics, e.g. tension of the shoulder girdle muscles in asthma.

General and Local Relaxation

General relaxation. Training in general relaxation is indicated in the treatment of psychosomatic tension states, and in the antenatal stage of pregnancy (mainly as preparatory training for the first stage of labour[1]). It is also used in the treatment of general postural defects and as a rest device in the treatment of patients by general exercises.

Local relaxation. Training in local relaxation is indicated in the treatment of such conditions as asthma, emphysema, ankylosing spondylitis and postural defects, where certain muscles are held in a state of persistent tension. The tension causes a muscular imbalance which, if unchecked, leads to adaptive shortening of the tense muscles and the adjacent soft tissues. Local relaxation training may be helpful in assisting the restoration of muscular balance and preventing adaptive shortening. General relaxation training is also sometimes used in the treatment of these conditions to counteract any general tension which may be present.

Where adaptive shortening has developed relaxation training is not indicated. Special exercises are employed which aim at lengthening the shortened muscles by activating their antagonists.

Relaxation in the treatment of lesions of the central nervous system. Specialized general and local relaxation training is employed in the treatment of certain lesions of the central nervous system, such as cerebral palsy. The aim is to achieve a temporary reduction of tension in the affected areas, so that re-education of movement may be attempted. This form of relaxation training is not discussed in this book.

REFERENCES

1. Heardman, H. Revised by Ebner, M. (1959), *Physiotherapy in Obstetrics and Gynaecology*, 2nd ed., Edinburgh: E. and S. Livingstone, Ltd.
2. Read, Grantley Dick (1953), *Childbirth Without Fear*. London: William Heinemann, Ltd.

Chapter 9

TRAINING TECHNIQUES

1. General Relaxation

The training technique used depends on the ability of the patient to relax his muscles consciously when he assumes a position which facilitates relaxation. The majority of patients for whom relaxation training is prescribed cannot relax their muscles satisfactorily, whatever the starting position used.

Patients who can relax consciously are trained to develop the sense of relaxation by practice in the position in which they can best relax. Patients who are unable to relax consciously are taught a series of exercises which induce general relaxation; the exercises are carried out as a preliminary to relaxation practice. In general, immediate results are not to be expected, and the training often extends over a period of several weeks. Regular and frequent practice on the part of the patients is essential for success.

Individual or class training. Relaxation training is carried out on individual or class lines. Class training often appears to give better results than the individual approach.

SECTION 1 : TECHNIQUES USED WHEN THE PATIENT CAN RELAX CONSCIOUSLY

Although the patient can relax consciously the therapist should explain to him the difference between muscular tension and relaxation. He is then taught the correct technique of positioning the body for relaxation (p. 73), and helped to find the position which affords him the maximum assistance in relaxing. At first (in addition to self-practice) he relaxes under the guidance of the therapist, who aids him by suggesting the sensation of repose in different ways. For example, he can tell him to think of giving up the whole weight of the body to the supporting surface, or of imagining the body to be so tired and heavy that it is falling like a dead weight through the mattress and the floor . . . Later, when the patient can relax without difficulty, he relies on self-practice alone.

Instructing the patient. The manner in which the therapist gives his instructions is of the utmost importance. His voice must be clear and distinct, but not loud, and the tone employed should be restful. The actual phrasing of the instructions should suggest repose, as indicated above.

The therapist's general bearing and approach to the patient is also important. He should have a calm and confident manner and be unhurried in his movements. When giving instructions it is advisable for him to stay in one part of the room and not move about, as patients who are practising relaxation frequently find it irritating if the therapist's voice reaches them from different aspects of the room. When instructions are not being given, however, the therapist may change his position if he wishes to do so.

Additional aids to relaxation. It is essential that the patient be warm and comfortable during the training periods. Before the training starts, restricting clothing, such as shoes, collars and ties, should be removed and the patients' attention drawn to the importance of emptying the bladder.

The room in which the training takes place should be as quiet as possible; if necessary, steps should be taken to shade the patients' eyes from strong sunlight or artificial light. In general, subdued lighting and restful colour schemes are not necessary, although in certain cases they may be useful.

Testing relaxation. During the training sessions the therapist should test the degree of relaxation obtained by the patient by passively moving his head and limbs. For example, he can lift one of the arms a short distance above the mattress, hold it in position for a moment or two, and then let it fall back unexpectedly into place again.

Sleep and relaxation training. Frequently the patient wishes to go to sleep during the relaxation session, and may actually do so in an involuntary manner. This is encouraged sometimes; for example, if the patient is suffering from insomnia as a symptom of a tension state. On other occasions sleep is not considered desirable during the relaxation period—e.g. when the patient is suffering from a general postural defect—as it interferes with his conscious approach to relaxation.

Concluding the relaxation session. At the end of relaxation practice the patient should sit up very slowly and rest for a minute or two before standing up. This gradual return to the standing posture allows for the alteration in blood pressure which takes place when the patient assumes the vertical position after being completely relaxed in a horizontal posture; it also "rounds off" the relaxation period in an appropriate manner. If the patient is allowed to jump up suddenly after practising general relaxation he may feel giddy and faint.

Use of music. Music of a suitable type is of value in helping the patient to relax. It may be used in each training session when the therapist has completed his teaching; it may also be used during the patient's self-practice periods. The patient is told to concentrate on the main melody and to think of nothing else.

A record player or a tape recorder is used; the volume control must be adjusted so that the music is just sufficiently loud to act as a soothing background to the patient's consciousness. If the volume used is insufficient the patient strains to hear the melody and ceases to relax.

Suitable music to use in relaxation training includes: *The Swan* (Saint-Säens), *Chanson de Matin* (Elgar), *Air on G String* (Bach), and *Largo* (Handel).

Positioning the Body for General Relaxation

Positions which facilitate relaxation are those in which the body is supported completely and the main joints are arranged in such a manner that their muscles are not stretched in any way. Five positions which fulfil these requirements are:

(1) Lying (Fig. 61).
(2) Modified side lying (Fig. 62, p. 74).
(3) Prone lying (Fig. 63, p. 75).
(4) Lying in full sling suspension.
(5) Half lying (Figs. 64 and 65, pp. 76 and 77).

Usually the patient prefers one of the positions to the others; the half lying position, when taken in a reclining armchair, is generally reserved as a progression on this selected position.

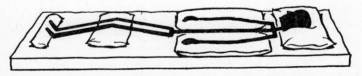

FIG. 61. Facilitating relaxation in lying. The feet are supported by a large sandbag; pillows are used to support the head, arms and legs.

Lying (Fig. 61). The patient lies on his back on a firm mattress, such as a spring, rubber or horsehair mattress, which supports the body without sagging. Pillows are arranged under the head, knees and arms, as indicated in Fig. 61. The feet are supported in mid-position by a large sandbag or foot-rest.

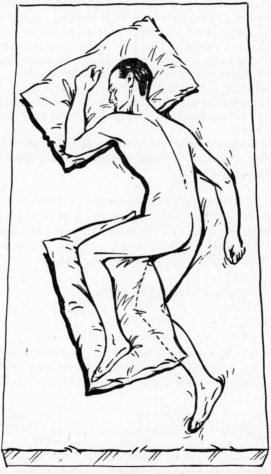

FIG. 62. The modified side lying position which is used in relaxation training. Note the oblique position of the head pillow, and the arrangement of the pillow under the uppermost leg.

The head pillow should be a soft one; it is arranged so that the cervical concavity is well supported. The arms are positioned with the shoulder joints slightly abducted, and the elbow joints flexed a little. The hands are supported with the wrists in the neutral position and the fingers slightly flexed.

Modified side lying (Fig. 62, p. 74). The patient lies on one side on a firm mattress with the trunk slightly flexed and turned towards the support, as shown in Fig. 62. The hip and knee joints are flexed, as illustrated, and the uppermost leg is supported by a pillow to relieve the hip abductor muscles of tension. The head is supported by a soft pillow, which is arranged *obliquely*, so that it also supports the uppermost arm. This arm is well flexed at the elbow and shoulder joints; the other arm is placed slightly behind the trunk as shown in Fig. 62.

Prone lying (Fig. 63). The patient lies face downwards on a firm mattress with the head turned to one side and supported by a soft pillow. A firm pillow is arranged under the abdomen and hips,

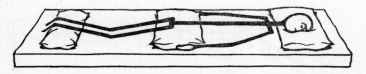

FIG. 63. The prone lying position modified for relaxation training.

to prevent hollowing of the lumbar spine and to flex the hip joints slightly. A third pillow is placed under the lower legs to flex the knee joints and prevent the toes from pressing into the mattress (Fig. 63). The arms rest by the sides, with the shoulder joints rotated medially and the palms facing upward; the elbow joints are slightly flexed.

Total suspension. This position is generally reserved for individual relaxation training. The body is fully supported by canvas slings, which are suspended from strong cords which run upward to an overhead frame; when correctly positioned the body rests a few inches above a bed, plinth or mattress. Springs are sometimes placed between the cords and the slings, or the cords and the overhead frame, so as to give buoyancy to the suspension.

The exact placing of the slings varies with individual requirements. In one arrangement which has been found of value the slings are placed under the following parts: pelvis, dorso-lumbar spine (including shoulder girdles), head, thighs, legs, arms and forearms. The feet and hands are supported by separate slings with the feet in mid-position, the forearms pronated and the wrists held in the neutral position.

The suspension cords are adjusted in length so that the knee and hip joints are slightly flexed, the spine kept straight, and the shoulder joints held in slight abduction.

Half lying (Figs. 64 and 65). The position is taken on a plinth or bed, or in a reclining armchair, as demonstrated in Figs. 64 and 65.

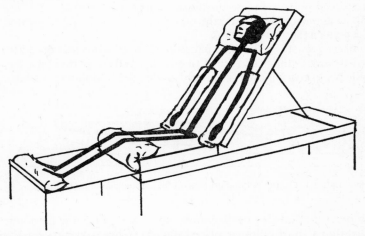

FIG. 64. Method of adapting the half lying position for relaxation training when a low plinth is used.

A soft pillow is used to support the head and fill in the cervical concavity. Sometimes it is found helpful to have two pillows, a small "sausage" pillow for the neck and an ordinary pillow for the head, as shown in Fig. 65.

Half lying on plinth or bed (Fig. 64). The arms are supported by folded pillows; the shoulder joints are slightly abducted, the elbow joints flexed, and the hands supported with the wrists in the neutral position and the fingers slightly flexed (Fig. 64). A pillow is arranged under the knee joints, and the feet are supported in the mid-position by a sandbag or foot-rest, as shown in Fig. 64.

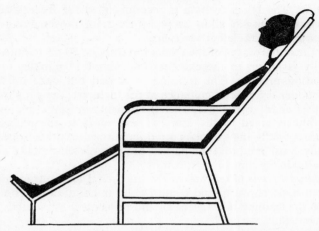

FIG. 65. Another method of adapting the half lying position for relaxation training: the position is taken in a reclining armchair. Note the small "sausage" pillow which is used to support the neck.

Half lying in a reclining armchair (Fig. 65). The forearms are supported by the chair arms, with the elbow joints flexed, the wrist joints in the neutral position, and the fingers slightly flexed; the shoulder joints are in a position of slight abduction (Fig. 65). If necessary, pillows are placed on the chair arms to cushion the forearms. The feet are either supported in the mid-position by a foot-support, as shown in Fig. 65, or rest on the floor.

SECTION 2 : TECHNIQUES USED WHEN THE PATIENT CANNOT RELAX CONSCIOUSLY

The therapist explains to the patient the difference between muscular tension and relaxation and instructs him in the technique of positioning the body for relaxation (p. 73). He then teaches the patient a series of exercises which help to induce general relaxation.

The exercises are carried out in the lying position on a firm mattress with the head, arms and legs supported in the manner shown in Fig. 61, p. 73. On the completion of the exercises the patient practises general relaxation in the same position, or in the modified side lying or prone lying position (pp. 74 and 75) if he has found one of these positions to be more restful than the lying position. The lying position is recommended for the relaxation exercises because it allows a wider range of movements to be performed than the other positions.

In the initial stages of the relaxation training 10–15 minutes are usually given up to the exercises and about 15 minutes to the relaxation practice. The training is carried out once or twice daily under the general guidance of the therapist; the patient also practises on his own. Later, when the patient can relax consciously, less time is given to the exercises and more to the relaxation practice; finally the exercises are discontinued. At this stage it is usually considered that the patient can rely on self-practice alone to maintain his control of relaxation.

Additional aids to relaxation. During the relaxation training the patient must be warm and comfortable; in addition the room in which the training takes place should be as quiet as possible. For further details, *see* p. 72.

Relaxation Exercises

The main muscle groups of the body are exercised in turn by a series of simple, small-range movements. With one or two exceptions the patient carries each movement to its limit, and then attempts to take it still further; he then slackens off the muscles completely and rests for a brief period. This combination of over-tension and rest not only produces relaxation of the muscle group concerned, but helps to induce a degree of general relaxation.

Any sequence of movements which is based on the principles of over-tension and rest may be used in relaxation training. A specimen list of exercises is given on pp. 79 and 80.

Teaching technique. The phrasing of the instructions and the manner in which they are given to the patient should suggest repose. The therapist's voice must be clear, but not loud, and should indicate the nature of the movements to be performed. For example, the instructions for the over-tension movements are given in a strong, positive tone, and those for the subsequent relaxation in a softer, more pliable tone which suggests a "letting go" or slackening off process.

The therapist's general bearing and approach to the patient should also contribute towards the creation of a restful atmosphere. He should have a calm and confident manner and be unhurried and restrained in his movements (*see* p. 68).

Specimen List of Relaxation Exercises

(Each exercise is generally performed 3–4 times in succession. An exception is made when the breathing exercises are performed, as indicated in the appropriate section.)

Legs

Movement	*Suggested Instructions*
1. Dorsiflexion of ankle joints.	"Bend up the feet . . . Pull hard!—harder! And let go . . ."
2. Plantar-flexion of ankle joints.	"Push the feet down as far as you can . . . Push harder! And slacken off the muscles completely . . ."
3. Inversion of the feet.	"Turn the feet in strongly . . . Further! And let them go . . ."
4. Extension of knee and hip joints.	"Straighten the knees as much as possible . . . Now press the legs down into the mattress . . . Hard!—harder! And flop out . . ."
5. Adduction of hip joints.	"Straighten the knees again . . . Press the legs together as tightly as you can . . . Grip hard!—harder! And let the legs roll apart . . ."

Arms

6. Extension of fingers and wrist joints.	"Straighten the fingers and pull back the wrists . . . Pull hard!—harder than that! And let go . . ."
7. Flexion of fingers, wrist and elbow joints.	"Bend up the fingers and wrists . . . Now bend the elbows fully . . . A bit more!—put every ounce of effort into it . . .! And let the muscles slacken off . . ."
8. Extension of elbow joints and fingers, with adduction of shoulder joints.	"Straighten the fingers and elbows, and press the arms against the sides . . . hard! Keep them there . . .! And let them fall apart . . ."

Head and Neck

9. Rotation	"Shut the eyes . . . Now roll the head slowly from side to side . . . It's heavy . . . and it's rolling easily . . . from side to side . . . Now stop, with the face turned forward, and rest . . ."
10. Flexion.	"Lift the head about an inch off the mattress . . . Hold the position! . . . and let the head drop back again . . ."
11. Extension.	"Press the head back against the mattress strongly. Harder than that! And slacken off the muscles . . ."

12. Temporo-mandibular joints and facial muscles.	"Clench the teeth together. Now 'screw up' the facial muscles very tightly . . . Tighter! And relax . . ."

TRUNK

13. Abdominal muscles.	"Pull in the abdominal muscles until they are quite flat . . . Pull a bit more . . .! And rest . . ."
14. Extensor muscles of the spine.	"Push the chest forward until you have hollowed the back strongly . . . Lift a little more . . .! And let go . . ."
15. Respiratory muscles. (i) *Very deep breathing*.	"Breathe in and out as deeply as possible . . . *In* . . . and *Out* . . . Force the breathing . . .! Deeply IN . . . and deeply OUT . . ."
(ii) *Deep breathing*.	"Now slacken off the breathing, and breathe in and out more easily . . . *In* . . . and *Out* . . . and *In* . . . and *Out* . . ."
(iii) *Normal breathing*.	"Breathe quite normally now, and follow your breathing movements with your thoughts . . . Concentrate on the breathing and put everything else out of your mind . . ."

N.B. Each of the first two forms of breathing is carried out for about 1–1½ minutes. Normal breathing, as a conscious exercise, may be performed for the same length of time or for a longer period, according to the benefit derived by the patient. Many patients find that they can relax better when they concentrate on the normal breathing movements.

Relaxation Practice

At the conclusion of the exercises the patient practises general relaxation in lying (Fig. 61, p. 73), or modified side lying (Fig. 62, p. 74), or prone lying (Fig. 63, p. 75). The therapist can aid the patient by suggesting the sensation of repose, as indicated on p. 71, and by employing suitable forms of music (p. 73). Music may also be employed during the patient's self-practice periods.

Testing relaxation. During relaxation practice the therapist should test the degree of relaxation obtained by the patient in the manner described on p. 72.

Sleep and relaxation practice. Often the patient wishes to go to sleep during relaxation practice. Sleep is encouraged in some cases and discouraged in others, as explained on p. 72.

Concluding relaxation practice. At the end of the relaxation practice the patient should sit up very slowly, and rest for a minute or two before standing up. If the patient jumps up suddenly after practising general relaxation in a horizontal posture he may feel giddy and faint (*see* p. 72).

2. Local Relaxation

Relaxation training for individual muscle groups which are held in a state of persistent tension (p. 69) is based on the techniques described in Section 2 of this chapter, and is not discussed here in detail. In brief, the patient performs one or two relaxation exercises which are localized to the tense muscles, and then practises conscious relaxation of the muscles.

The training is carried out on individual lines with the body completely supported so that none of the muscles is stretched in any way; particular attention is paid to the positioning of the joints controlled by the tense muscles. Suitable positions include lying (Fig. 61, p. 73), half lying (Figs. 64 and 65, pp. 76 and 77), and lying in full sling suspension (p. 75).

Example of training technique used to relax tense pectoral muscles. From a suitable lying position the patient rounds his shoulders as much as possible—attempts to take the movement still further—and then slackens off the controlling muscles completely and allows the shoulders to drop back to their original position. He rests the muscles for a few moments, and then performs the exercise again. During the rest period he attempts to "let go" with the pectoral muscles.

The exercise is performed about 10 times in succession under the guidance of the therapist (*see* p. 78 for Teaching Technique); the patient then practises conscious relaxation of the muscles for a period of about 5–10 minutes.

At the beginning of treatment supervised training is given daily, or twice daily, and the patient is encouraged to practise on his own. Later, he relies on self-practice entirely.

Relaxing the muscles in sitting and standing. When the patient can relax the pectoral muscles satisfactorily with the body fully supported, he should be taught to attempt the relaxation techniques in the sitting and standing positions, without the shoulders being supported in any way. In this manner he learns to acquire the habit of relaxing the muscles in normal circumstances.

Indirect Local Training

Localized relaxation of tense muscles is sometimes achieved in an indirect manner by general exercises. For example, to relax the muscles of the shoulder girdle, rhythmical arm swinging exercises are used. During the swinging movements the therapist lays stress on the importance of letting the shoulders move in a relaxed manner, but does not teach a conscious relaxation of the muscles.

Chapter 10

SO-CALLED PSYCHOSOMATIC TENSION STATES

By

MAURICE PARSONAGE, B.Sc., M.B., F.R.C.P., D.C.H.

Consultant Physician to the Neurological Department in the General Infirmary at Leeds. Senior Clinical Lecturer in the University of Leeds. Consultant Neurologist to the Leeds Regional Hospital Board.

Introduction

It has for some time been recognized that a sizeable proportion of chronically sick individuals suffer from long continued aching pain which appears to be related to a state of persisting abnormal tension in their body musculature, particularly that of the limbs and spinal column. Moreover, numerous careful observations made by investigators interested in this problem have led to the view that such a state of abnormal muscular tension is an integral part of a general state of excessive and unremitting nervous tension which develops insidiously and may pass unrecognized.

The notion that a muscle or group of muscles may become the seat of aching pain seems not unreasonable when it is recalled that such pain may develop in a normal individual if he subjects his musculature to prolonged activity, as, for example, when he indulges in unaccustomed exercise. Under such circumstances the involved muscles soon become the seat of pain and tenderness both of which may endure beyond the period of active muscular contraction. In the case of the chronically anxious and tense individual it appears that much of his bodily musculature may exhibit persistently increased tension, as if in preparation for motor activity which is either inhibited or does not find a satisfactory outlet. The muscles of such individuals can sometimes be felt to be abnormally tense when examined and sometimes the presence of increased activity can be demonstrated and measured quantitatively by electrical methods in precisely those muscles which are the seat of chronic aching pain.

There may thus be some justification for the recognition of what may conveniently be termed a psychosomatic tension state or syndrome and in this chapter an attempt will be made to give some account of how these states may arise, how they may manifest themselves and how they may be treated. Their importance derives from the fact that they are of very common occurrence in medical practice; furthermore, the treatment of such conditions may be difficult, since it involves a special approach and technique which places considerable demands upon the patient, as well as upon those who are treating him.

Psychological Aspect of the Problem

Abnormal states of tension in body and limb musculature may arise under a variety of circumstances. They may on the one hand be quite local in distribution and are then often related to underlying bone or joint disease. In such cases the muscular tension or spasm is regarded as being largely protective in function by virtue of the fact that it serves to immobilize the diseased part. On the other hand the abnormal muscular tension may be more widespread, and it is then more often found to be related to a state of abnormal nervous or emotional tension to the development of which consideration must next be given.

The emotions of fear and anger appear to be of outstanding importance from the point of view of the development of psychosomatic tension states. These two emotional states are of fundamental biological significance since they spring from the instinct of self-preservation and when aroused by an appropriate stimulus normally lead to purposive action. This results in dissipation of the nervous energy which has been accumulated in association with the arousal of the emotion. In the animal kingdom at large threats of danger to life serve as the natural stimuli in arousing these emotional states which become the effective driving forces in the development of a state of preparedness for action—flight from danger in the case of fear, or a more aggressive or self-assertive reaction in the case of rage or anger. In either case widespread bodily changes take place which are concerned with mobilization of the energy reserves of the organism in preparation for intense muscular activity. Modern man has inherited this same pattern of response to danger from his ancestors, although important modifications have naturally occurred with the development of civilization and accepted codes of behaviour. Yet we can still recognize the utilization of this primitive instinctual behaviour pattern in action in, for example, the case of the athlete at the commencement of a race. At this moment his mind and body are geared to a state of readiness for violent muscular activity which has been brought into being by the arousal of feelings of competitiveness (self-assertion) and fear lest he fail or do badly in the race. However, the moment the starting signal is given his accumulated nervous and bodily tension is transmuted into appropriate action, which is then normally followed by a period of rest and relaxation when depleted energy stores are made good.

Important modifications in the state of an individual are, however, likely to develop when for some reason appropriate action cannot follow immediately or reasonably soon after the arousal of a given emotional state. Thus, in the case of fear a state of anxiety and dread supervenes when action is impossible, or a state of sullen anger (resentment) when aggressive impulses have been aroused and cannot be expressed. These states will of course tend to persist until some means of discharging the accumulated nervous energy can be found. For reasons which will later become apparent this may be a matter of very great difficulty for an individual and he will then be liable to develop the symptoms and signs of psychosomatic tension syndrome. Consideration must therefore now be given to the circumstances under which such states of inhibited (frustrated) fear or anger may arise.

The Anxiety of Everyday Life

In dealing with the circumstances in which anxiety (frustrated fear) may arise we may consider first what might be termed the anxiety of everyday life. This occurs when an individual is involved in a worrying situation such as the threat of severe financial loss, illness in the family, threatened loss of prestige, and so on. Here the fear is due to an obvious outside cause and must be endured until such time as the situation may change. If the individual is of a sanguine disposition the anxiety is unlikely to reach serious proportions but if he has a nervous disposition, perhaps as a result of his having been exposed to seriously disturbing experiences in childhood, then the degree of anxiety shown is likely to be considerably greater. This is so because latent fears, often induced by early childhood experiences, now reinforce or augment the present anxiety, making it appear excessive when considered only in relation to the recently developed circumstances. But anxiety may also arise when the threat of danger comes not from without but from within ourselves. Thus an individual may distrust his ability to control his own temper or keep his natural aggressiveness in check. Fears of this kind are apt to produce anxiety because the individual cannot escape from himself; however, if he recognizes and is conscious of the source of danger, then this usually proves to be an important mitigating factor.

It frequently occurs, however, that the source of anxiety in an individual may be quite unknown to him since it stems from some portion of his mind of which he is not conscious. Because the source of the fear or anxiety is unconscious and hidden it is beyond the control of his will and cannot lead to appropriate action. It is then termed neurotic and the subject may in these circumstances be suffering from what is known as an anxiety neurosis. Such a sufferer exhibits either a generalized vague persistent fear of almost everything; or he may become anxious or even panic-stricken when alone, or in an open or a closed space, and he is then said to suffer from phobias of one kind or another. It seems to be the case that in many anxious, tense individuals the anxiety originally stemmed from exposure to fear-producing circumstances in infancy or childhood. These are multifarious and include illness, nurture by a mother of anxious disposition, threats of or actual separation from the mother, ill-treatment from parents, frequent parental quarrels, exposure to terrifying experiences and feelings of deprivation of love. Such circumstances as these do not, of course, necessarily always lead to the development of neurotic fears and anxiety later in life; yet they are, nevertheless, likely to act as predisposing factors, since they are apt to be re-awakened when the individual is subjected to stressful circumstances in later life. There are a number of ways in which the child attempts to deal with the anxiety or fear induced by his early experiences, although there are perhaps two which are of foremost importance from the standpoint of this chapter.

Defence Mechanism

In the first of these reactions the fear eventually undergoes an automatic removal from the conscious to the unconscious portion of the mind, a process technically known as repression. It is then commonly replaced by an attitude of independence and self-sufficiency which may then become the child's permanent dominant characteristic. What has happened is that the child, without knowing it, has erected a kind of barrier or defence against his fear. So long as this barrier remains intact the consequences will not be serious but if it is broken down all the old fears may then emerge, resulting perhaps in some form of nervous breakdown. Nevertheless, children who develop a defence mechanism of this kind often grow up to be men and women who are hard-working, energetic, efficient, conscientious, ambitious and usually successful. Yet this is at the expense of an underlying state of strain and anxiety which is ever likely to spur them on to greater and greater efforts, thus tending to make them habitually tense and unable to relax. There is therefore a pre-disposition to breakdown which may finally be brought about by some precipitating cause such as family worries, business reverses, and so on.

In the second type of reaction to early childhood fears a process of repression again occurs in favour of an attitude of self-assertion ; but this now assumes a more pronounced form of aggressiveness (self-will) which is apt to be associated with feelings of hate and resentment when there have initially been feelings of deprivation of love. A further development then commonly follows in which the self-assertive attitude is itself displaced in favour of a more docile, moral attitude whereupon the individual comes to fear his own aggressive impulses. This is termed the obsessional type of reaction and is of great importance from our present viewpoint, since it is commonly met with in individuals who develop psychosomatic tension syndromes.

The Obsessional Type of Individual

The outstanding characteristic of the obsessional type of individual is that, despite an outward semblance of docility, he is liable to be assertive, self-willed and defiant. He feels impelled to have his own way and to dominate, but the fear of his own aggressiveness compels him to adopt an attitude which often makes him appear dependent, over-anxious to please and even timid. There is thus a conflict between his strong self-will on the one hand and his exaggerated fear of the consequences of its expression on the other. The latter is essentially a moral fear and not one of objective dangers in the face of which such individuals are normally courageous and sometimes seemingly fearless. This conflict between self-will and the fear of the consequences if it should be freely expressed is, of course, very common in childhood; yet it is a conflict that can be solved in a variety of ways, by no means all of which may be at serious cost to the individual's development and stability. If the child has been endowed with a basically aggressive temperament he may simply become defiant and rebellious, character traits he may well be able to turn to good account under favourable circumstances. On the other hand, if the fear of consequences is strong and he is of a more docile temperament he may then grow up to be accommodating and amenable without apparent detriment to his self-assertive impulses. It seems to be only when the self-will and fear of consequences are both strongly developed that the obsessional type of reaction is likely to occur.

The obsessionally constituted subject is basically an anxious and insecure individual because of his fear-producing childhood experiences, and it is these that predispose him to be morbidly afraid of his own self-assertiveness. This fear becomes more intense when the latter is strongly developed, either because he is constitutionally aggressive, or because his basic self-assertiveness has become unduly fostered as a result of an injudicious up-upbringing. At all events the child, because of his fundamentally anxious nature, feels that he must constantly curb his aggressive self-will in order to secure the affection or acceptance of those with whom he lives and associates. During the course of his development he acquires what is known as a strong super-ego, which is the psychological term used to describe those reactions of the personality which are developed in response to the demands of the social environment. The super-ego is in fact that part of the personality which is essentially concerned with social and moral values. It is highly developed in the obsessional individual in whom it serves as a strong deterrent to the expression of aggressive impulses or tendencies.

Types of Obsessional Reaction

In the severer types of obsessional reaction various distressing nervous symptoms may eventually make their appearance, particularly if the individual is exposed to unfavourable circumstances. For example, if the fear element is predominant he may fall a prey to irrational anxieties in which a persistent fear of harm befalling himself is pre-eminent. If, on the other hand, the self-assertive element predominates then he may find himself constantly threatened by the emergence into consciousness of aggressive impulses, with the result that he has a persistent dread that he may do harm to others. Reactions of this kind, as well as others which will not be described here, comprise the various types of obsessional neurosis and fall essentially within the province of the psychiatric specialist. We are here more particularly concerned with a much less severe form of this type of disorder in which the moral super-ego is the dominant feature. In cases of this kind the individual strives to keep his aggressive impulses in control by adopting an attitude which is distinguished by the exhibition of what are known as obsessional character traits. Such individuals are constantly pre-occupied with the necessity of being absolutely scrupulous and are apt to be excessively conscientious in everything they do. Unfortunately this involves a certain rigidity of character which makes it difficult for them to adapt themselves to changing circumstances. Such individuals accept as normal their exaggerated and unduly rigid moral standards; moreover, they have a strong urge to maintain them at all times, even at great personal cost, because only by so doing can they feel acceptable to themselves as well as to others.

Obsessional Character Traits

Obsessional character traits are in fact of widespread occurrence but vary considerably in degree. We are here, however, mainly concerned with those milder examples in which the general attitude displayed is one which has been aptly described as perfectionistic. In such cases the general picture is one of a basically insecure individual whose social adaptation depends upon a constant striving to live up to such maxims as the necessity to be always prompt and orderly, to keep one's feelings to oneself and never lose one's temper, to be always absolutely truthful and to owe nobody anything. In any given individual the emphasis may be upon any one or more of these various attributes, although it will be found that in many examples of this type of personality structure no one particular aspect is developed to an extreme degree. Although this outward attitude is in fact a defence against the emergence of aggressive impulses, to the casual observer it will appear to be essentially a constant striving to be perfect. Of course, such an urge, if not unduly strongly developed, can often be put to good account, because such individuals are likely to be good, reliable, conscientious workers who can fulfil an important rôle in society.

Unfortunately the perpetual striving towards the maintenance of what are only too often unrealistic standards is apt to impose a considerable amount of strain upon the obsessionally disposed individual. Such a pattern of behaviour is moreover very likely to lead to frustration and disappointment when circumstances are adverse and the standards demanded by the super-ego can only be met by an ever-increasing effort. This then seems to be the general sort of setting in which psychosomatic tension states are especially likely to develop and consideration may now be given to their characteristic clinical manifestations.

CLINICAL MANIFESTATIONS

In many instances it will be found that sufferers from psychosomatic tension states consult their doctors initially on account of persisting aching pain and stiffness which is characteristically felt at the back of the head and neck, across the back of the shoulders and in one or more regions of the spine. The pain may often be, in the early stages at least, relatively localized to the back of the neck or the lumbar region of the spine for varying periods of time. Nevertheless, it has a marked tendency to become more widespread and not infrequently it may radiate down the limbs also. In most cases it appears to be essentially related to the musculature, and the patients will often report stiffness and tenderness of muscles which are especially the seat of pain. Sometimes patients are aware that there is an abnormal degree of tension in their muscles, especially when the tension is experienced in the muscles at the back of the neck where it may give rise to a sensation as if the head were being pulled backwards. It is characteristic of the pain in general that it is apt to persist for days, weeks and even months at a time. Sometimes it tends to worsen towards the end of the day and it is apt to become intensified when the patient has extra difficulties to cope with. Characteristically, it is only temporarily relieved by the simpler pain-relieving drugs and by ordinary physiotherapeutic methods (massage, radiant heat, etc.).

Types of Head Pain

Various types of head pain are common. Frequently this is felt at the back of the head and appears to be extending upwards from the back of the neck. At other times it is felt across the forehead as a dull ache, over the top of the head as a sense of pressure or like a weight on the head, or as a tight band encircling the head. Typically, these varieties are also persistent for long periods of time and are relieved little if at all by the simpler pain-relieving drugs such as aspirin or codeine. In contrast to head pains of this type many sufferers will be found to complain of paroxysmally occurring headache which frequently proves to be of migrainous pattern. This is a throbbing form of headache which is usually localized and mild initially but soon increases in intensity and may become widespread as it does so. It may often be confined to one half of the head and is not infrequently associated with vomiting and prostration. Particularly characteristic of this type of headache is its liability to occur shortly after or in the wake of a period of increased activity or stress when the patient might normally be able to relax his efforts, as at weekends. Although it is generally accepted that the mechanism of this type of head pain is a painful dilatation of extra—or intra-cranial blood vessels, there is much to suggest that mounting nervous tension, particularly when the emotional state is one of suppressed rage, can often bring this mechanism into action. Lastly, mention should also be made of the fact that some of these sufferers, possibly a significant proportion, seem liable sooner or later to develop sustained high blood pressure, a complication the significance of which is still not properly understood.

Other Symptoms

Many of the patients will also complain, or admit on direct questioning, of feelings of tenseness, restlessness and difficulty in relaxing. Such symptoms as these comprise the general background of the disorder and, although they vary considerably in intensity, they are often of sufficient severity as to make falling asleep at night difficult. Usually further questioning will reveal evidence of the underlying state of emotional tension and this commonly assumes the form of either an all-pervading anxiousness, or of an obsessional striving to maintain unrealistically high standards, as has already been described. In many cases the operation of environmental stresses will be evident. The importance of these cannot be over-estimated and their rôle must, of course, be carefully appraised. Even so, time and again it will be found that it is the patient's own inner attitudes which are a major source of difficulty; however, the detailed evaluation of these is essentially part of the treatment process and will receive further consideration later.

Physical Examination of the Patient

The findings on physical examination are not as a rule remarkable. The difficulty these patients have in relaxing their muscles may become clearly evident when they are asked to lie on the examination couch. Sometimes those muscles which are complained of as being especially painful may be observed to be abnormally tense when an attempt is made to stretch them passively. Broadly speaking, however, the general physical examination of the various bodily systems is usually productive of negative results, except when the situation is complicated by an abnormally raised blood pressure. Nevertheless, the whole physical examination must be carefully and systematically carried out in all cases. This is necessary in order to exclude as far as possible the presence of underlying organic disease and not merely to impress the patient with the thoroughness with which his case is being investigated; nevertheless, the latter is a matter of some importance, as experience in the treatment of these patients has clearly shown. Lastly, it should be mentioned that in many instances it may also be necessary to employ various laboratory investigatory procedures before an adequate total assessment can be made. Thus, an X-ray examination frequently proves to be indispensable, particularly when problems arise with regard to the assessment of such commonly associated factors as cervical and lumbar spondylosis.

PRINCIPLES OF TREATMENT

If the rôle of emotional factors in the production of the various varieties of psychosomatic tension syndrome be acknowledged it would seem to follow that perhaps the best policy would be to refer all such cases to the specialist in psychiatric disorders. The large number of these sufferers alone would make such a policy somewhat impracticable, but there are other reasons to be taken into consideration. Perhaps most outstanding of these is the fact that with few exceptions these patients are very strongly biased towards the view that their symptoms are of wholly physical origin; this need occasion no surprise when it is realised how commonplace is such a belief and that their general upbringing and outlook naturally incline them to take a very organic view of their disorders. They are apt to feel, too, that there is something disgraceful in suffering from a complaint in which "nerves" appear to be the principal offenders. Moreover, their natural unwillingness to accept such a possibility has only too often been enhanced by the purely physical treatment which has so frequently been meted out to the vast majority of these sufferers in the initial stages. It will be quite clear therefore that referring these patients direct to a psychiatrist will be very apt to arouse their antagonism, a difficulty which may be a serious or even insuperable bar to effective treatment. It is in fact the authority of the organically oriented physician that is so very necessary in the handling of these patients whose confidence and active co-operation must be secured at the earliest possible stage.

First Stage of Treatment

The treatment process begins from the very first moment the patient and doctor come into contact with one another. The initial history-taking and physical examination of the patient comprise the foundations upon which the later stages of the treatment are based; the thoroughness with which they are carried out will do much to win the confidence of the patient which the doctor must ever be at pains to secure. In practice it may be found convenient to take the patient's history in the conventional manner and then proceed at once to the physical examination. It can then be decided whether or not any investigatory procedures, X-ray examinations, etc., are necessary, and when these have been dealt with a preliminary assessment of the case can be made. At this stage the problem can usually with profit be discussed frankly with the patient and the proposition put to him (or her) that nervous or emotional factors are in all probability playing an important rôle in the production of the illness. Usually the patient will be found to be willing at this stage to countenance such a possibility, provided that the initial physical examination has been systematic and thorough. The doctor must also make it quite clear at the outset that he accepts the genuineness of the complaints and recognises the patient's very

real need of assistance, as well as the subconscious or unconscious origins of the disorder. The observance of this latter
proviso is essential to the establishment of a satisfactory thera-
peutic relationship with the patient, even though it may demand
much skill and patience on the part of the doctor.

Second Stage of Treatment

The next stage in treatment consists in the taking of a very
much more detailed history of the development and course of the
patient's illness, relating these wherever possible to the events and
circumstances of his everyday life. In this way it will often become
clearly apparent, both to doctor and patient, how the latter's
experiences and attitudes are intimately bound up with the
occurrence and intensity of his symptoms. An individual suffering
from a psychosomatic tension state should have no very great
difficulty in understanding at least the rudiments of such a
relationship, given average intelligence and a reasonably good
ability to co-operate satisfactorily. The essential purpose of this
stage of the treatment is to increase the patient's insight into his
condition. However, it must be emphasized that in the type of
case now under consideration this does not involve intense
probing into the patient's mind or the use of complicated psy-
choanalytical techniques.

The Doctor's Rôle

The doctor's rôle is essentially one of teacher, counsellor and
friend. His first task is to assess critically the history as com-
municated by the patient, to explain to him as far as he can how
the symptoms have come about and to give him some understanding of the psychological and physical factors which are their
underlying cause. This is usually not a matter of great difficulty,
but the process of re-education which follows will usually be
accomplished far less easily, particularly since it may demand
much of the patient. The aim at this stage is to help the patient
obtain a better understanding of himself so that he can appreciate
the doubtful value of such qualities as orderliness and accuracy
if they are unrealistically applied so as to lead to inflexibility and
frustration. In this way the patient may eventually learn sounder
and more efficient methods of handling his difficulties with results
that can hardly fail to be beneficial.

The principles of treatment dealt with so far have been mainly those concerned with psychological aspects of the psychosomatic tension syndrome. They have received prior consideration because of their prime importance in the programme of treatment and they should always precede the employment of physical treatment of any kind. This is so because the patient cannot be expected to co-operate willingly and intelligently when physical therapy is applied, or derive maximal benefit from it, until he has a reasonably clear understanding of the nature of his illness. The psychological approach is therefore the sheet anchor of treatment and will usually need to be applied in one form or another throughout the whole of the time the patient remains under medical care.

Relaxation Therapy

The physical treatment of choice which is to be combined with psychotherapy in dealing with patients suffering from psychosomatic tension syndromes consists of a course of instruction in muscle relaxation exercises. The technique of this is described in detail in chapter 9. It is here therefore only necessary to emphasize the fact that their essential purpose is to teach the patient to relax his over-tense muscles. When he has learned to do this satisfactorily he is enjoined to make use of the technique for as long afterwards during the course of his everyday life as may be necessary. In the early stages at least it is often helpful to combine the administration of muscle relaxant drugs with the teaching of relaxation exercises and allowance must be made for the fact that some patients may at first experience some increase in their sense of uneasiness as they begin to make progress with their muscle relaxation. This latter effect may not be inconsiderable but it should not often be a serious obstacle to the continuance of treatment since it can usually be overcome by judicious handling of the patient. In some cases the patient may fall asleep when carrying out the muscle relaxation exercises and experience has shown that this may prove to be a valuable acquisition, particularly when insomnia has been a troublesome feature of the illness.

CONCLUSION

Experience has shown that muscle relaxation exercises can be effectively applied as an adjunct to treatment in a variety of nervous disorders in which anxiety and tension are outstanding.

Many of these, however, may be of a serious nature, such as the severer forms of anxiety state and the anxiety occurring in association with schizophrenic and depressive illnesses. Such conditions as these come wholly within the province of the specialist in psychiatric disorders and are entirely beyond the scope of this chapter.

The considerations which have been here discussed apply essentially to the milder forms of nervous tension which are met with in the less severe anxiety and obsessional states in which persisting abnormal muscle tension is a prominent feature. These are conditions which are so commonly encountered in hospital and outside medical practice as to demand the attention of doctors practising medicine in many branches other than that of pure psychiatry. The term psychosomatic tension state or syndrome has been adopted simply as a convenient diagnostic label, since it serves as a perpetual reminder of the importance of taking into account both psychological and bodily factors when dealing with disorders of this kind. Our understanding of these and other types of so-called psychosomatic disorder is still incomplete and it may be that with the growth of knowledge in this field it will ultimately be possible to apply more satisfactory and precise diagnostic labels.

The results of treatment by the method which has been outlined in this chapter are difficult to assess. Even so, experience so far has indicated that they are likely to be more satisfactory than those obtained when physical methods of therapy alone are used. Sometimes the difficulties encountered in the treatment of sufferers from psychosomatic tension states may be considerable. For example, it may be found that more is demanded of the patient than he can apparently give, with the result that some disappointments and failures will be inevitable. Perhaps, therefore, the most that can be expected of the combined psychological and physical approach which is here recommended is that a substantial amount of relief from symptoms can in all probability be obtained in a sufficient number of sufferers to justify the trouble and effort. Furthermore, the results of such treatment are likely to be more enduring than would be the case if a less comprehensive approach were to be adopted.

ACKNOWLEDGEMENT

I remain indebted to the late Dr. D. R. MacCalman, formerly Professor of Psychiatry in the University of Leeds, for his helpful advice and criticism in the preparation of this chapter in its original form in 1956.

INDEX

99